Mindfulness of a Fly on the wall

A journey to mind, body and soul

By

Mansfield Grey
(Stephen Gregory Brown)

Stephen Gregory Brown

This book contains the opinions and ideas of its author. It is sold with the understanding that neither the author nor the publisher is engaged in rendering financial, legal, consulting, psychological or other professional advice or services.

Mindfulness of a Fly on the Wall
by Mansfield Grey
a Sunao International publication
Copyright © 2018, Stephen Gregory Brown

Cover by Matthew Many

Printed in the United States of America. No part of this publication may be reproduced, stored in a retrieval system, or transmitted in any form or by any means, electronic, mechanical, photocopying, recording, scanning, or otherwise, except as permitted under Section 107 or 108 of the United States Copyright Act, without the prior written permission of the Publisher, or authorization through payment of the appropriate per-copy fee to the Copyright Clearance Center, MA 01923.

ISBN-13: 978-1719221085   ISBN-10: 1719221081

First Print and Ebook Editions July 2018
Stephen Gregory Brown 1961 -

10 9 8 7 6 5 4 3 2 1

SunaoPublishing.com

sunao

Mindfulness of a Fly on the Wall

Contents

Mindfulness of a Fly on the wall 1
    A journey to mind, body and soul 1

Contents 4

Book One 6

Chapter 1 7
    The Day of Awakening 7

Chapter 2 16
    Mind 16
    What Is Consciousness? 16

Chapter 3 22
    What is Ego? 22

Chapter 4 34
    Changing The Way You Think? 34

Chapter 5 38
    Is your glass half empty or half full? 38

Chapter 6 42
    What is Conditioning/Programming 42

Chapter 7 51
    Ego's Mask 51

Chapter 8 67

The Life Puzzle 67

Chapter 9 70
What Is Mindfulness? 70
Practice creates calm 70

Chapter 10 80
Soul 80
What is Self Actualization? 80

Chapter 11 89
God and the Devil 89

Chapter 12 92
Discipline of Mind 92

Chapter 13 102
Energy of Life 102

Chapter14 107
States of Consciousness 107

Chapter 15 115
Re-Conditioning Yourself 115

Chapter 16 119
Live in Excellence 119

Chapter 17 123
What is Our Purpose 123

Chapter 18 133
Body 133
Physical Fitness, ... 133
Time to Awaken Your Vessel 133

Chapter 19 .... **144**

    Neuro Gravity Resistance Lifestyle 144

Book 2 .... **161**

Accounts of a Fly on the wall **162**

    (It Was What It Was) 162

Parents, Asthma, and "Make That Second Effort" **163**

Building Integrity **172**

The Only Marilyn I Ever Knew **178**

Sports and Consciousness **182**

Arnold, Lou and the Flipper **189**

Layers of Life **199**

If I can get it for you in blue, would you buy the car? **205**

Love, Ego, and "I am not one of those guys' **213**

Florida, Forklifts, a Smile and A lotta Cars, ... **222**

This Life, Findings and Observations **236**

I Am, The Fly, Now **247**

Mansfield Truths: **249**

    THE END 249

Book One

Stephen Gregory Brown

Chapter 1

The Day of Awakening

My name is Mansfield Grey. There was a time in my life when I was in my forty-fourth year. I was married for the third time, had three adopted kids and three step kids. I had worked at many different jobs and careers and I was always changing women, friends and surroundings. I look at it now and see all the different lives I have had.

I think of all the groups of friends I have been blessed with, those who have come and gone in my life. Some have died, some have lost touch, and others have been lost and then re-connected after years of non-contact. Most have moved on with their lives, as I have done myself many times.

One morning, as I was deep in thought about this very subject, I heard a voice. I didn't know where it was coming from. I looked around the kitchen and no one was there. Where was it coming from?

I couldn't make out what it was saying, but it sounded like a faint whisper in my ear.

The only other living thing in the room was a fly. It seemed to fly a little, then sit for as long as I was in that room. I dismissed it and went about my day.

The next day, while getting ready for work, I heard that faint whispering in my ear again; a little louder, but I still couldn't make out what it was saying.

This seemed to happen on a regular basis for a while. I would hear the whispering a little louder each day. As per usual, during a Canadian summer, there were always flies to be found buzzing around our house. We have four dogs and a cat and were always going in and out of the doggie door.

Then I began to hear the voice whispering in my ear while away from home. I thought I was going crazy: The voice wouldn't stop. It kept getting louder each day. It was driving me crazy until one day, while I was making my lunch in my kitchen, I saw the Fly for the first time and I heard a voice scream at me loud and clear.

The only thing in that room was me and a Fly. I looked at that Fly and asked in a sarcastic way, "what do you want Fly"? and I laughed...then the Fly answered.

Fly:

I am the Fly. I am *your* Fly, here, now. I will be with you from now on. I have always been and will continue to be, a Fly on your wall: Listening, watching, and feeling. You can't get rid of me. I will be there. I am not what you think I am. I am not a voice in your head you have been hearing, that has been getting its own way for so long. I am not "the justifier"; "the logical one"; "the man's man"; "the warrior,"; "the barbarian." The one who is the judge and jury. Hah! No! I am not him, nor am I the one who you think you are. These are all ideals on which your thinking, up until now, have taken place.

I watched you become a star hockey player, a track star, a basketball star, a competitive bodybuilder, retail sales clerk, roofer, construction worker, material handler, gym membership salesman, car salesmen, business machine salesman, Industrial products salesman, forklift sales, car sales, professional actor, personal trainer, and a truck driver for a beer company.

I have watched your life unfold to have countless lovers, wives and girlfriends.

I have witnessed your life as a father figure for six children; three step children and three adopted children. I have watched how you helped raise them all and become a part of their lives. I have watched how you have always led with love but have gotten caught up in all the wave of consciousness and drama so common to North America.

I have witnessed your melt downs, your weaknesses, the embarrassing moments and the trials and tribulations of your life.

I have watched you learn to be the pack leader of four dogs and a cat.

I am here to set you straight on what you have learned in life to this point. I am here because you want me here. You asked me for help. You knew I was always here but didn't know where. You weren't sure if the feelings you had and the voice you heard were real.

I am the Fly. I have always been the other one in your mind that would let you know that. "Your time will come, be patient,"

Do you remember that?

Mansfield Grey:

I have always thought that *my time would come.* That was you? I didn't know what that meant. I thought I was being weak, making excuses for not succeeding at the time.

Growing up my father instilled in me the "Vince Lombardi" principles. He hung them from a mobile on my ceiling in my bedroom. I would awake each morning with these quotes being the first thing I saw when I woke up:

Winner's never quit and quitters never win.

Mental toughness is essential to success.

Fatigue makes cowards of us all.

Make that second effort

Winning isn't the everything, it is the only thing

Fly:

Yes, I have seen your whole life unfold. Sometimes a lot of confusion, emotion and strife, but all-in-all you are a pretty calm person. Those "Lombardi" principles you learned when you were young have stayed with you throughout your life. You hated them then, but later realized you loved them.

I am here now to help you make sense of it all.

Mansfield:

Why are you here? How can I hear you?

Fly:

I am here because you are awake from your sleep now. You have done everything *your* way up until this point in time and you are not happy. You have been successful in so many things, but still can't find peace in your world. I am here because you asked for a better way and you are awake and being true to yourself. You do know when it all started to happen, don't you?

Mansfield:

When I broke up with my second wife and lost my job in the same month it really blew me away. It made me think: *Is this, what life is? Is this it?* It sucks! There has to be a better way? That was when I hit bottom.

Fly:

I knew, but you didn't hear me back then. That's when you started to awaken. It takes a long time to find the true you, and accept it, embrace it, and love to live with it. That was your start. You have come a long way. A long journey that is your journey, and only yours.

You are a very independent person; always have been. You like your space. You like to be with yourself, just as you have been conditioned to do so with your asthma when you were young. You like alpha consciousness, you prefer it. You are creative, loving and positive. You are good energy.

Mansfield:

If you have been here the whole time, seen all I have done, thought, tasted, felt, smelled, why didn't you say anything?

Fly:

I did, you just weren't listening. You knew me when you where young. Asthma was our common thing. I was always there with you when you couldn't breathe. I helped you concentrate on every breath for survival, for hours at a time. I am the one who helped calm you down, manipulate your body's energy, the one to open your lungs, so you could breathe. I worked alongside your wonderful mother, who would scratch your back to ease the tightness in your chest. You didn't know, but I taught you to meditate to relieve your asthma, concentrating on every breath: In and out, in and out, until your breathing was normal again. Your mind became conditioned to meditate in those tough times at age four. You learned at a young age to find alpha consciousness.

This has helped you through your whole life, by having to come back to the moment and concentrate on now. Concentrate on your breathing. You have always had this ability, but thought it was all normal and everyone with asthma could do it.

Then they came out with the asthma puffers, and fifteen seconds later you where good to go. Over the years as you grew, my voice faded into the background, but when it counted you heard me and he took credit. You listened to the other voice in your head most of the time. The "BOSS," the "EGO". He was the good guy to you back then and he is still here. He is just losing his power because you have had all the Ego experiences you could have imagined when you were a kid. Now there is nothing left for your Ego. Ego is bored. It wants something better. Now is the time to evolve into the next consciousness. It takes a long time. It takes a lot of work. But you are on your way.

Chapter 2

Mind

What Is Consciousness?

Mansfield:

What is this new Consciousness? Do you mean "*how you think*"?

Fly:

Yes, how you think. Your consciousness is most important of all; it affects everything that takes place in the body. How you think is directly related to how the body functions. Which is: It protects from disease, heals fatigued systems, converts fuel to energy, and disposes of waste products.

When we analyze our consciousness, we often forget that what the mind thinks, the body will follow. In this busy world, we get caught up in all the drama, finances, schedules, deadlines, commitments, appointments, dates, plans, experiences, future, and past. What's going to happen? What happened? How has it affected me? Where will I go from here? What do others think of me? What do I think of myself?

All this and more create chemical reactions within the body. These chemical reactions can be a positive thing or a negative thing. Stress can be a good thing if conditioned right. It can be minimized, but it can't be eliminated. When we get stressed, the body goes through changes and adapts to what it needs to, to ensure survival at that moment. In doing so, the body produces cortisol to deal with the increased heart rate, increased blood pressure, increased body temperature, which in turn can make you feel nauseous, head ache, tired, sweating, etc.

When the body produces cortisol, it must dispose of the hormone when the stressful situation has passed. It must be filtered through the liver and excreted out of the body in a few different ways. It does this by defecation, urination, via the respiratory system and the sweat glands. The central nervous system is a well-oiled piece of machinery, which ensures survival at all costs.

When a stressful situation happens, our consciousness is the thing that determines if that situation is actually stressful or not which is based on past experience. If there is no past experience, then the situation could be elevated to an even more stressful event. In some or most of these situations, the experience can be trained or conditioned, allowing us to deal with the same stressful situation and have minimal hormonal changes within the body, giving the whole system a break. In turn the mind adapts and the body follows through conditioned training.

Mansfield

What should the ultimate goal be for a human?

Fly:

The ultimate goal is consciousness that has mind, body and soul, as one and have the ability to stay in that state for long periods of time, absorbing positive energy from the universe and live in joy, internal peace and gratitude.

Mansfield:

How do we attain mind, body and soul, as one?

Fly:

That is a question with an answer that is complex. In order to achieve mind, body and soul, as one, it takes a lot of work, reconditioning of the psyche and mental awareness, or mindfulness of one's self. The goal here is to find absolute control over the Ego, to the point where Ego and self mould into super Ego alone, taking over the ship or vessel. This means control over all emotions all the time.

This absolute state of mind: self actualization, has been labeled by a scientist named Maslow. He named his study of human motivation: "Maslow's Hierarchy of Needs. "

He believed there were eight levels of how humans motivate themselves. These are learned behaviours that help humans achieve what they want.

He believed that we are first motivated by our biological and physiological needs: air, food, water, shelter, warmth, sex and sleep.

After these needs have been met and learned by Ego, Ego then moves on to level two, which is safety. The need for the human psyche to feel security and protection from the elements, are all natural physiological needs that date back to the beginning of human kind.

Level three is "Love and Belonging". The Ego craves intimacy, trust and acceptance. It searches for the ability to give and receive affection and to empathize and belong to a group, work, club, etc.

Level four is "Esteem". This is the Ego and what it experiences, how it learns to acquire the physiological needs, the safety needs, and the love needs. It is the level of motivation that defines a person's self worth, while being unconscious of their thinking.

Level five is "Cognitive Needs". This is the pursuit of knowledge and understanding, curiosity, exploration, the need for meaning and predictability.

Level six is "Aesthetics". This is the search for and appreciation of beauty, balance and form.

Level seven is "Self Actualization". This the ultimate goal. When self and Ego become aware of each other and meld to become one. This level is where one realizes one's own potential, seeks personal growth and self fulfilment. Where creativity shines.

Level eight is "Transcendence". This is when the need to help others reach self actualization.

Maslow noted that only one in a hundred individuals ever get to self actualization because society only rewards level one, physiological needs. Therefore, one could become literally stuck in a pattern of trying to attain these rewards by following a conditioned pattern that Ego has learned earlier. They become lost in their own Ego, over and over again.

If you become mindful of your own Ego you can change the patterns and move toward self actualization. Remember, Ego is always involving in every waking moment of your consciousness.

Chapter 3

What is Ego?

Mansfield:

Explain what Ego is?

Fly

Ego is the Greek word for "I". This is your fear center. This is where the boogie man lives and is just around the corner. Watch out! Ahhh, he missed you again, huh?

Ego is the voice inside your head that tells you what to do based on previous patterns, learned or conditioned. Self is the feeling you get when you know what the right thing is to do. Often we follow the Ego because that's our conditioned or programmed state of mind. As a child, Ego loves instant gratification, the quick reward, the big payoff, the end of journey. Or so we think.

Ego is usually giving the least amount of effort possible, with the biggest payoff: The "What's in it for me?"
or: "I don't deserve this…woe is me!"

Ego complains whines and cries about anything. Ego is the excuse maker when tasks are unsuccessful. Ego always has its back up, waiting for someone to attack, so it can be ready to defend and conquer. The battle plays out in Ego's head over and over. Always success or always failure. These are the patterns of the Ego that repetitiously play until self realizes this is only your conditioning.

The Ego spends lots of energy on the future and the past. It whines and cries about past events that draw sympathy or, on the other side, the Ego shouts at the top of its lungs how great it is and it needs to show everyone else how great it is too. Once Ego shows the world how great it is, it will then, and only then, be happy.

If people are being born every minute all over the world, it will be an endless journey for Ego to show how great it is. There will always be one more person to impress.

Ego can only live in the future or in the past. It is bored in the present. It needs to be entertained in the present. It needs to be fed in the present. It needs to grow in the present. Then Ego is our greatest ally and our worst enemy.

Learning how to control Ego is what our journey here in the material world is. This is what Jesus was teaching so long ago. He was teaching people to control their Ego. It is what could change humanity forever, if the consciousness of all was the same. The energy we could produce would be remarkable. We would have "Heaven on Earth".

If you can be aware of Ego, you can learn to control it and therefore control your health by keeping stress level hormones low, allowing the body to function at a higher level. This makes it more efficient in healing from exercise, food assimilation, deeper sleep, and strengthening the immune system.

Cortisol (stress) retards the functions of the body. It is like a hostile enemy attacking the vessel from the inside. The body must process these negative hormones and try to somehow excrete them. The best way to get rid of cortisol is to exercise. The more core oriented the exercise is, the better.

Ego is to blame for stress because stress is a man-made creation. Each and every one of us has our own and separate reality that we are living. We can choose any way we want to lead our lives. Why are so many of us not happy, not satisfied and complaining about it...always wishing tomorrow would be better? Hah! That's your Ego.

Realize it and change it. That is up to you. Once you have some control over Ego, you will begin to see the real picture out there in the world, if you don't already.

Everything is geared toward self gratification: "The child that wants it now!"

At the same time the Ego is a child that is scared deep down and wants to fit in. It is wanting everyone to accept it. This is what humans have to deal throughout their lives; trying to manage their Ego's.

The conditioning of society's psyche is created to live in an Egotistical world that drives the engine of the machine we call the economy. It is an Ego-generated machine that needs more and more and more. It will never be satisfied.

"If I only had more, I'd be satisfied." That is the state of the world today, as a Fly sees it.

The Ego will never be satisfied. Satisfaction means death to the Ego. It needs the future and dwells on the past. It is labeled and recorded for the Ego to recall in another similar experience. And used again.

The Ego also loves to worry, especially about situations, other people and things it can't control.

It plays scenarios in your head, pictures of disaster, failure, and rejection. The "I don't deserve to be so happy." It is a saboteur.

These feelings you get from all the negative energy hurts the body, creating havoc with digestion and sleep. In actual fact the collective consciousness of EGO, if not controlled, will kill the human race through uncontrolled emotion of the masses.

Mansfield:

What happens to Ego once self-actualization has been realized?

Fly:

If you are lucky enough to get to self-actualization you will see the big picture. You will realize your full potential for what it is you are here on this earth to do at this particular time and that can change in time due to more experiences.

You, Mansfield Grey, have experienced all that is needed for Ego to evolve into finding more self-fulfilling activities to become more creative and desire your own personal growth.

All the old is a "been there done that" kind of thing. All old things that use to entertain you are now boring. Creativity is your new motivation. You do things for yourself, not for a reward. You don't go around telling people what good you have done to get an Ego boost of "What a good person you are". You have integrity. You are the same person when people are looking, as you are when they are not. You no longer feel you have to play roles anymore, although you are quite capable of taking them on. Basically, Ego takes a back seat and changes places with true self.

Ego was educated through your experiences and conditioning, then self takes that knowledge of training and uses it to be the driver of the vessel now. The vessel being your body.

Mansfield:

Can we eliminate the Ego?

Fly:

The Ego will always be there. You need it for survival in this material world. But it needs to be recognized and controlled. You need the Ego to make sure you are not being taken advantage of. You need to be aware of Ego being detrimental to health as Ego can cause numerous illnesses. Again, what the mind believes the body will follow.

Mansfield:

How can we control Ego?

Fly:

Jesus taught truth. Jesus taught about Ego even before Sigmund Freud defined it and what it does.

"Deny thyself!" Jesus said. He was talking about Ego. Deny what the Ego wants if it is attained with conflict between Ego and self. Therefore, discipline is what Jesus taught.

If you deny the Ego, or have your Ego in line with true self, the "do the right thing" mind set, then the body benefits with non-destructive physical reactions within the body.

Less stress is beneficial to the body. It keeps the blood it in a more positive PH level and keeps the immune system working at optimum levels.

Once you become aware of Ego you can start to control your actions, thus controlling your health.

To control Ego you must control your emotions. In any given situation you should respond to the situation and not react emotionally. Emotions create energy, responding is control. Reacting is volatile uncontrollable emotional energy that is given out with no control. Leaving the body to recover and try and process all the stress chemicals that are detrimental to human health.

Mansfield:
What creates stress?
Fly

Sigmund Freud, who theorized his Id, Ego and super Ego theory back in the early 1900's stated that we are all a product of our conditioning and most mental disorders can be cured if we can find how the subject's conditioning of the past experience related to the present experience. The two experiences could be completely different, but very similar by just analysis.

Id is instinctual survival needs: food, water, shelter, sex, love. The Id objective is to survive at all costs.

The id needs Ego for survival. The Ego is in control and Id works in accordance to what Ego wants.

Ego decides how you will obtain these survival necessities. Once these needs are met, the Ego then develops and grows based on experiences of how the survival needs were attained and continues its' conditioning. It categorizes the past, it envisions the future and decides what we will be.

Super Ego (or what I would call true self) limits decisions based on law, conditioning and morals. What is taught as right and wrong.

When you are born and start to develop your Ego, the Maslow's Hierarchy of Needs discussed earlier, is where the Ego finds what is successful and what is not in attaining the physiological and behavioural needs. From that conditioning on, the Ego will use these experiences to attain the physiological and behavioural needs as it has before, defining the procedure of attaining and labelling for the next time it is required to attain these needs. This is what motivates you.

All these decisions are made in the frontal cortex of the brain. It self regulates and gives the ok first, i.e.: Does it break any rules of society? Is this experience morally right?

Ego steps in and starts to rationalize all possible outcomes, wanting to be satisfied in the future, wanting and rationalizing that we as a whole (the body) will be better off than now, after we attain and go through that experience. Ego can convince self to go along, even if it isn't morally right or unethical.

Everyday, all day, the Ego is the leader or captain of the ship. The ship being the vessel we call us (our body). Ego is driving the ship.

Is your ship broken? Do you feel tired, weak, unmotivated? What is your next move? Are you excited in anticipation, or are you dreading tomorrow? Are you enjoying right now?

The Ego cannot live in the now. Now is boring for the Ego. The Ego must be entertained. The Ego must have a purpose. The Ego has to have everything labelled, defined, judged, then stored in the memory as good or bad. The Ego will never be satisfied with now. There will always be something missing and the Ego will work hard to find and label what is missing so it can go back to work to make it better. This is an endless cycle never to be actualized.

When events are experienced and not planned it just happens as life does and you feel it is a wonderful moment. You do not realize it when the moment is happening. You realize it upon reflection of the experience. It is then more defined and labelled by the Ego and placed in the memory. Human conditioning of the

Ego trains us to re-enact the same experience to try to find that good feeling you had from the first time you experienced the event. As you notice, you can never go back. You can never create the same spontaneous feeling you had when the original experience happened. Something is always missing. The spontaneity is gone because Ego has planned the whole re-enactment.

It is like seeing your favorite band play in concert. You see them the first time and WOW! Second time wow! Third time wow. Fourth time you think maybe you don't have to see this band again, even though you are still a fan. It is a "been there, done that" scenario. Ego says.... Next!

The reason seeing the band isn't a WOW! anymore is because the Ego has experienced this before and needs to be entertained with something else... something better. No matter how the Ego will try to rationalize why you should see that band again, it can't find the satisfaction and energy it got the first time you experienced this band in this moment with this person, on that day, with how you physically, emotionally and spiritually felt. It was a moment, and each moment is its' own. It was and always will be. Ego always wants to be in control of the destiny and wants something better than the last time.

An example of this is in the mass consciousness of western society with the way entertainment has evolved. It is an "anything goes" mentality. Thirty years ago you couldn't swear on television. Today nothing is off the table and the more shocking the better. The Egoic consciousness of society has pushed the envelope on entertainment. The Ego always needs to be entertained.

Chapter 4

Changing The Way You Think?

Mansfield:

Ok, but how can you change the way you think?

Fly:

What if you could condition your Ego like you condition your body with fitness? What if you could control hormonal changes with the exercise you do, the food you eat, the sleep you get and the water you hydrate with? These are all things we can control.

We can control the way we think. Therefore, we can control the way our body functions with the right kind of training based on science and evolution.

Can you imagine your world with very minimal stress? We create stress for ourselves because that's what the Ego wants. The Ego needs to live in turmoil, drama and anxiety. Ego uses negative emotion: anger, pride, envy, revenge, jealousy, laziness, etc. to justify our means. It destroys the body in the process by opening up negative energy patterns that change the electromagnetic field of the body to receive and process that negative energy current throughout the body. You will feel this physically by way of your emotions. It is very physically exhausting dealing with these emotions along with the negative chemicals the body produces.

This will happen if Super Ego is, or self is, in conflict with Ego. Ego will always try to silence the self. Self is the "goody two shoes" who is hiding deep down. Ego locks it in the basement and will only let it out when no one is around.

Problems and high stress occur when Ego is oblivious to self. It has hidden self in the basement so long it has become acceptable to self.

Ego lives in fear that true self will be revealed and status will all be taken away: (Maslow's Needs). It lives in fear that identity of who they have classified and labelled themselves as will be truly revealed.

When Ego is threatened it becomes offended. This happens whenever you feel disrespected or wronged. That is Ego jumping in to protect self from not being taken advantage of. Ego will use emotion to get the offence dealt with. With offended emotion comes stress. With stress comes worry which creates cortisol. An insecure Ego gets offended a lot. If Ego gets offended a lot then there is bad stress hormones racing through the body, weakening the immune system and promoting disease within the body.

The Ego hates change. It is an unknown about the future and unclassifiable. The Ego cannot live in the now. When you feel you are bored, that is your Ego, because now is not where Ego wants to be. Ego wants to be engaged in something that will make the future better or trying to re-enact the past for entertainment or self loathing. If you are bored, it is not you that is bored, it is Ego. Ego cannot be now and Ego needs to know what is to come tomorrow because it has already defined, classified, slotted, planned, and imagined tomorrow a thousand times.

Once the Ego has done that, classifying tomorrow, the Ego decides: Is it good or bad? This is where some individuals have difficulties. Ego is always analysing everything in reference to how it will affect you.

Chapter 5

Is your glass half empty or half full?

Fly:

The pessimistic, half empty approach, is going to produce cortisol as worry, anxiety, and depression, which will set in until the experience is over. Then Ego will dissect every bit of the experience and tear it and your own character apart.

The optimistic, half full approach, is going to produce small amounts of cortisol, only when thinking directly about the up-coming event, or what just happened. This allows you to control how much you think about the same stressful event, therefore minimizing cortisol.

Half empty, the mind remembers all bad outcomes, feeling all of the pain of an unsuccessful event as if it actually happened. Cortisol shoots through the body, along with gobs of adrenaline, keeping you from sleeping and making you worry, likely causing you to fail because of your own self-fulfilling prophecy, or "Ego- fulfilling prophecy". What the mind believes the body will follow.

Again, everything is based on past experience. Someone who has done the same event many times is going to produce less cortisol than someone who has no experience at the same event, even if the experienced person doesn't like what the event is.

The mind, Ego, plays a major role in the health of the human body. It controls not only external interactions, but internal functions of the various systems that make our bodies (which are really the biological machines that we drive.) function.

Mansfield:
When or how do we get our Ego?
Fly:
That comes from our conditioning. We are all born with the self. Ego starts to develop the minute you come into this world. From being given a name and identity, a space

in this world, Ego starts to develop by mimicking what is perceived.

You as a one-day-old baby are given a blanket. This blanket becomes "your" blanket. And as you grow, that blanket becomes "my" blanket. Me, I, myself, are all statements that say "I am an individual and I own that blanket". "That is mine". You also subconsciously mimic whoever is around and spends time with you. If it is your mother, she rewards you with a smile, a facial gesture, a laugh.

The Ego then records the laugh, smile, tones, and mimics them. When this happens, mom rewards you with her love and happiness. This continues with all different people and experiences throughout your life. You start to mimic those people who Ego perceives to be successful. Conditioning always changes throughout your life and you learn to mimic from birth.

As you grow, you become educated in this monetarily run, Egoic world we live in. Ego, being developed in every experience, from brushing your teeth with *my* tooth brush, to writing an exam and finding out what *my* mark. Ego's conditioning questions:

"How does *my* mark compare with the rest of the class?"

"How much do *I* really care about this mark and class?"

"How will this mark affect *me*?"

"What will others think of *my* mark on the test?"

This is how your Ego develops when growing up. Each experience is dissected and evaluated to be good or bad and it is labelled to be a part of you until you can realize that the conditioning of your Ego is really not the true you.

The true you is inside, just as it was when you were an innocent baby and got your first blanket and were told it was yours. The true you has no words. Words are learned by the Ego. Your true self, you, has no words, it is just a feeling. Ego describes what you feel. Ego deals with the material Egoic world. Ego is there to protect self.

As you develop your Ego, the Ego eventually takes the place of the people who raised you, trained you, made you think that way. We are all products of our conditioning until we realize that the way we were conditioned is not one's true self.

Mindfulness of a Fly on the Wall

Chapter 6

What is Conditioning/Programming

Mansfield: What do you mean conditioning?

Fly: Conditioning is the way you were educated into this world from day one. Whether you had two parents who loved and cared for you, nurtured you until you left the nest, or no parents and left to raise yourself. Your conditioning is how you perceive the world to be, while driving your vessel, the body. It is all your experiences up to the point when you realize you are not your conditioning. It is all the rules, etiquette, mannerisms and identities you have taken on, what you think you are to others and what you perceive as good or bad. It is all your judgements and categories you place things under. Your feelings and actions are all from your conditioning from day one. When you said your first word, that was conditioned by your Ego growing and your consciousness growing. When you said your first words you where rewarded with positive energy from your mother or father or whoever was present.

You were told "Good boy for saying Momma".

You unconsciously noticed you liked how this positive energy felt coming from momma and you wanted it again, and again, and again. Then your Ego got bored of that energy as it couldn't be satisfied with that same reward. So Ego wanted other words to say and get rewards. And off the Ego went craving more reward, more challenge. And when each challenge was met, your self esteem grew. Your Ego grew.

Everyone has a different conditioning. When you realize you are not your conditioning, is when you start being aware, or mindful of your Ego.

This is why there is so much turmoil between countries, religions, people, and races. They believe they are their conditioning and do not realize that is why they think the way they do. They were programed to think this way by the culture they have identified with. They think they are their Ego. They are unconscious.

When Ego's conditioning is threatened by what it believes is right, it fights back with negative emotions like anger, jealousy, and contempt. Ego wants to stand up for its' conditioned beliefs and will die trying, as in the case of war. This really does happen.

Mansfield: When is my conditioning complete?

Fly: Conditioning is complete the moment you realize you are not your conditioning. You are now aware of your conditioning and now the journey starts; the re-training of your previous conditioning.

On the physical side of things, conditioning takes place within the brain until the early twenties. The brain and mind are forging neuro pathways through experience that make us who we are for the rest of our conditioned life. Once conditioning is realized, then and only then can the process begin to re-condition the mind into molding self with Ego.

It would be as if Ego is there to protect self, until self is ready to take over and run the show: Drive the ship, steer the vessel. Ego is still there, it is just morphing into a version of self, aware that it is now a team effort. Ego will still refer to old conditioning periodically simply by habit.

Some humans never realize throughout their lives that they are a product of their conditioning. That is how they have been conditioned and it does not reflect who they really are. It is just what they were taught and how they continue to act to the point where they become their conditioning.

You know all about conditioning, already. I am just here to put your puzzle together.

Mansfield: What do you mean I already know about conditioning?

Fly: You know everything I know, you just can't see it yet. But the picture is clearing.

You have lots of experience with conditioning. You studied psychology in school, so you learned about Freud and Pavlov's dog and experimented with behavioural conditioning with wild pigeons. You have always had three or more dogs and cats that you had to train and be a pack leader. You also raised three adopted children from ages six to ten years old. You help raise three step children starting when they where nine years old, with different conditioning than the others. You have watched how various conditioning changes from family to family and how it impacts the lives of these children as they grow.

The conditioning of your children, or should I say the re-conditioning of your adopted children, was fascinating to witness. The kids came to you at ages six: a boy, and two girls ages eight and ten. They came from a family of neglect. The father had issues and ended up in jail, while the mother would sometimes take off for days at a time, leaving the ten-year-old daughter to care for her younger siblings. No school, nothing. They were on their own till mom came back.

When they would play, the oldest would make the younger ones play her games and bully them into playing, sometimes by pinching the others and using violence, mimicking what she had witnessed.

These children were conditioned by their parents for this kind of lifestyle. They came into your home like robots. They all moved as one, from one room to another. They would always compete with each other for everything. The oldest girl was always relentless because she was the pack leader and she usually got to be first, got the first thing, bullied her way through, but she was the mother to her siblings. She was the main care giver to her brother and sister. If something went wrong when mom was gone, she was to blame. She shielded the younger two.

You and your wife had to re-condition the children from Day One. They were six, eight and ten and they didn't know how to comb their hair. They didn't know how to reply when someone said "good morning" to them. They had to learn everything, I mean everything. But first they had to try, which was some days impossible. The only words they knew were "I can't" and they used those words a lot. They were so afraid of failure because the conditioning they had was very negative in energy, verbally abusive and sometimes physically abusive, from the birth parents. They had no self esteem. They had not had a loving family to help condition their behaviour and teach them how to try, let alone love.

The great thing about adopting children from Children's Aid is that you need to be approved, go to classes on what to expect from a child who has been conditioned poorly, and wait for a child that would fit into your family. In other words, a good match.

The first thing you needed to do with the kids was come right out and in a loving calm assertive way, tell them you were their parents now and that you will love them as they should be loved. You and your wife told them to do as you say because it is for their own good.

When someone says "Good morning" you say "Good morning" back" and all three, in a chorus, said "ok".

You never had a problem again. They just were never taught simple things like that.

That's where you had to start from. It was a twenty-four hour a day job and the great thing about it was they all wanted to be taught. They wanted to be told what to do, what the rules were. They never had any rules before. They were just yelled at and punished when something was unacceptable.

You also had to get them to find themselves within. They had grown up as a threesome, protecting each other for survival. Like three wild animals that were just trying to survive on popcorn and soda. The three kids had only one personality. It was a group consciousness based on the oldest one's interpretations of what happened. She would dictate the others reactions. They would copy her.

The cure for that was to re-condition them to be individuals and yet still be part of a bigger group. You had to do activities with each child individually, re-enforcing that their opinion mattered and it was ok to think differently than the others. All the while still correcting their behaviour and telling them how to act in situations that would come up. In other words, the parents are now the pack leaders as they should be and the kids are there to learn about life and be conditioned to fit into society securely and smoothly.

A good example of conditioning is a story your oldest daughter told you once when she was sixteen. She told you of time when living with her birth parents, both parents where home and got in an argument. The father got so mad that he kicked the family cat down the stairs and killed it, right in front of the kids. He made the kids clean up their dead pet and place it in a garbage bag and take it outside. As my oldest daughter was about to pick the cat up when her younger brother, who was only two years old, walked up to the dead cat and started kicking it, to mimicking the father. He wanted to be like dad. He was being conditioned to behave this way toward another life.

If your son never left that home, there is a good chance he would be in jail or dead by now.

Now the kids are all grown up and living happy lives. All the hard work, classes and educating ourselves with what was needed paid off.

Ego is the product of your conditioning and its job is to protect self and survive.

Stephen Gregory Brown

Chapter 7

Ego's Mask

Mansfield:

How does Ego protect me?

Fly:

We all are trying to portray a certain image, build our self esteem and fit in. Ego will decide who you are and what role you will play. Ego will pick the best mask it can find, so self won't be discovered. It goes for something that will make self and the vessel (the body) stand out yet conform with peers. It could also go to the other extreme and want to be different. An individual. The individual is the rebel from society, but wants to be noticed. It loves the attention but doesn't know it. It wants people to think they have it all together, but in actual fact, they are more insecure than most. These are the bully's, the mean girls, the people that need to be talking all the time so no one will say anything derogatory, because they can't get a word into the conversation. These are just some masks people wear, and roles they play to hide their true self.

Mansfield
What is a Mask?
Fly:
A *mask* is an image that Ego wants to portray to society and their peers. A mask would be something like many tattoos, piercings, bodybuilding muscles, latest fashion, nice car etc. Masks can also be behaviours such as getting into trouble with the law, arrogance, laziness, complaining, gossiping.

Basically, a mask is a superficial role being played while Ego keeps self safe. That mask is made up of all previous experiences and Ego picks the best experiences of the past and what it wants future experiences to be. The Ego picks the image of self.

You, had an experience when you where in grade five which had a lot to do with the mask and role you have played up to now.

It was 1976, you were ten years old you where one of the class leaders in school. You had lots of friends. Sport was your passion. Especially hockey. You were naturally talented to play and your father was a great teacher of the game.

One afternoon in class, you where getting a lot of attention from everyone while the teacher was speaking. You where being disruptive to the other students in the class.

One student said to you to "shut up and be quiet".

He embarrassed you and you said to your-self, "How dare this little whimp say that to you!"

You where having your moment stolen. You got really pissed off and told him to meet you after school by the fire hydrant where you wanted to teach him a lesson. You where only ten years old and you where threatening another student like you saw them do on TV.

A full forty-five minutes goes by and school is out. You can remember when the bell rang to be excused from school. You consciously thought that you didn't want to fight. You knew you could take him easily, but you also knew that you had to get out of it and do it in a way that all your peers would still respect you. After all, in a fit of anger forty-five minutes ago you promised you would beat the poor guy up. Now with a cooler head, you had to follow through to be the tough guy, but you also knew you could never purposely hurt anyone. That is because self would not let you, for that is your true nature, but Ego couldn't let it go. You continued to play the role of the bully, even though you didn't want to. Your reputation was at stake.

You came up with a great plan to purposely get a detention, so you would have to stay later than the other kids and you would be able to avoid having to beat this poor kid up.

In a fit of rage, your Ego challenged him and condemned him and when Ego calmed down self stepped in and didn't even want to fight. Self just wanted to go home and get some eats.

The poor kid I am talking about is the guy everyone picked on. He was different. Liked different things. He kept to himself a lot. He was definitely weaker than you.

You thought it would all just go away, but oh no, all the guys had to try and stop him from leaving school grounds until you were out of your detention. Now you had to beat him up just because you said you would. You had an obligation and didn't want to go back on your word. That's what Ego was saying in your head.

As you exited the school after your detention, your pals were waiting.

"Ahh!" they said. "He got away and ran into the principal's office. He told the principal on you. You're in trouble".

You went home worrying all night and dreading school the next morning.

The next day came and you were called down to the office. The principal explained to you about threatening and bullying. He told you it was wrong.

You already knew it was wrong and hadn't wanted to do it in the first place, but this was the role and the mask that you were wearing at the time school was let out.

You had to apologize to the kid you were bullying and serve two weeks detention. You promised the principal that you would never do it again.

Mansfield:

Yeah, I remember by the time school was over, I had calmed down and began to just play the role of a bully. I didn't want to hurt anyone.

Fly:

Ego was in charge of the moment when the kid talked back to you. Ego thought it was a challenge and reacted. Masks and roles were then drawn and your true self/super Ego didn't want to participate. You even remember telling the principal that you would have never hurt him. You just wanted to scare him.

That is Ego. The student you wanted to beat up was weaker by far, but Ego wanted to exercise its' power over him in front of all your friends. This was all negative energy.

What Jesus says about that is "What you put out you receive twice as much back" and you got it back being bullied two times in your life after that incident.

The first time was not long after you were the bully. It was a cold winter day and you and your buddies were playing road hockey out front of your house.

This local hood was riding his bike up the street with a friend. You had known him from school. He was a rebel and everyone was afraid of him. He was three years older and used to go to your school just the year before. You and your friend admired this kid. He smoked cigarettes, acted cool like he didn't care about anything and was always having a good time at other people's expense. He was a bully.

Mansfield:

The previous year we would always bum cigarettes off of him to be cool like him. Looking back, I remember a moment in time when he was riding the opposite direction we were walking.

As he drove by he asked, "You guys want the rest of this smoke?"

"Sure" we replied.

He then dropped it in our hands as he sped by and we smoked it. We had hung around the convenience store many times with him and we thought he was our friend.

I guess not, because that cold winter morning he walked up our street as we were playing road hockey. He and a couple of other bad kids were acting up as they approached.

He came right up to me and asked. "See this egg, would you go running to your momma if I broke this on your head?"

I was trying to be tough and said "No"

So he broke it! Right on my head, in front of all my friends and started to laugh. I swung my hockey stick at his shins and started to cry. My pride was hurt because I had egg running down my face and was frustrated because he was bigger and could beat me up if he desired.

I ran in the house to tell my mom. I was devastated emotionally.

I guess that is what is meant by, "what goes around comes around".

Fly:

That was the first time you got bullied. The second time was when you were in grade seven.

You where bullied by a bigger, older student from another school over a girl you had not spoke to, or seen, in six months.

He was a hired gun, asked to beat you up because his friend's girlfriend, who you had a relationship with earlier in the year, still liked you. So you were to be beat up over something you had no control over.

You were now the bullied and you didn't like it one bit. You were stressed.

Anxiety and worry, all part of your days for about two weeks. Until you decided that you wanted this to end because you could not live like this anymore. It physically hurt, worrying all the time.

You confronted the bully one day after school. You knew you would get your ass kicked but wanted to stop worrying and stressing over it.

In front of everyone of your peers you submitted to him and said "I will not fight back, I know you are stronger, bigger, and older. You explained that it wasn't your fault if his friend's girlfriend still liked you. You had no intentions on her; you hadn't had any contact in months.

He accepted what you had said and didn't beat you up. He let you go.

From that moment on, you decided that you would never let anyone have the opportunity to bully you again.

This experience is where your choice to wear the mask and play the role of a bodybuilder originated.

You thought "If I am big enough, no one will ever pick on me again."

"Do you remember that?"

Mansfield:

Yes. I do but hadn't thought of that for years.

Fly: This was a major decision in your life to develop your specific Ego and self esteem and it has affected you for your whole life. This mask you wore is but another small piece of your puzzle. It enabled you to play the role of bodybuilder for thirty-five years. You knew if you where different from others, you might stand out without having to say much. It protected you from bullies and enabled you to support yourself through acting, because you where a bodybuilder. You where trying to mimic Arnold Schwarzenegger.

Mansfield:
Does Ego always have the same mask?
Fly:
The mask is always changing throughout one's life. When you become aware of Ego and all that it has done or hasn't done for you, good or bad, the masks start to come off slowly. Still shy, very guarded is self. But awareness of Ego is the key.

You have changed your mask so many times, but always kept the mask of bodybuilder. You were a salesmen/ bodybuilder, personal trainer /bodybuilder, roofer/bodybuilder, actor/bodybuilder, truck driver / bodybuilder, father/lover/brother/son/bodybuilder.

You will always have bodybuilding in your realized conditioning because that has benefitted your health your whole life. The fitness will continue to be a part of your life until you die, because it is so engrained in your psyche.

You have chosen to keep this part of your conditioning, because it is a health benefit to the body. Your training with weights has become unconscious to the point of creating new neuro pathways to muscles you weren't previously aware of. And it continues to expand and grow bringing mind, body and soul together.

The bodybuilding has been a major part of your life because it actually taught you discipline of the Ego. Deny thyself from unhealthy foods, not enough sleep, low hydration, bad Egoic emotions. These would be all detrimental to building muscle within the body.

Psychologically your thoughts were, maybe you can make some money being a big actor like your idol *Arnold.*

Like the time when you first started acting on camera at age thirty. You had developed your Ego to the point that you had been playing all these roles throughout your life. So, the next thing you would try was acting. No training, only a few classes you thought to yourself, or Ego thought. You were going to be a guy who plays the role of an actor auditioning for parts on film, television and commercials. It all was a role, but not the real you. You never showed interest in acting as a kid or adult, why now? Well, turns out it was all an Ego thing, all about the money and attention from others.

The first time you auditioned you where so nervous you could barely say your name. The nerves are the Ego, not wanting you to look like a fool in front of others. It was the Ego's conditioning of protecting self from hurt feelings or embarrassment of being found out that you were not really an actor. Or were you? That is Ego. As you continued to audition, it got easier and easier until you got your first speaking role on a series.

Mansfield: Oh yeah, "Due South".

Fly: Yes! That was a crazy time for you. A major moment in your life.

At thirty-one, you had auditioned and secured the role of goon. It was an actor role. So that meant you got paid more and you had eight or less lines. You knew your lines inside and out. It came down to rehearsal and blocking the scene, which was in a jail cell. Paul Gross, Calum Keith Rennie and two great character actors were in the cell opposite you. You were the goon that gets thrown into the opposite cell of the two bad guys. They were playing the parts of Van Zant (aka Al Waxman) the mob boss' henchmen.

The Director was George Bloomfield. He says "Action" for the rehearsal and you draw a total blank?

Oh my God, you think to yourself.

All the blood drains from your head and it feels like you're about to faint.

Mansfield:

The feeling of failure came over me. I was in a panic. I was feeling small and intimidated. I felt this way once before and the outcome was not good.

It was when I was in junior hockey. I was the captain of the team and we were playing for the championship. The team we were playing was intimidating and big. I was the biggest guy on my team and believed in my mind that I was the guy that had to stick up for all my teammates.

Fly:

The only thing was, that you were a skills player, you weren't a fighter. That moment in time wore away on true self back then and was a major conflict in life for Ego and self. So much so that the stress made you sick with flu like symptoms for the last three games of the best of seven series.

Your team lost in overtime in the seventh game and it was a big failure in Ego's eyes. Ego thought you were a failure for not being who Ego thought you should be.

It wasn't in self's true nature to be the goon or bully. You had great anxiety for days.

Now you had your first speaking role in television and you couldn't remember your lines. It made you have the same anxiety, the same physical feelings, as you had playing in that hockey series all those years ago. Ego was having a meltdown.

Mansfield:

I had to compose myself and deliver my lines! NOW! Or everyone would find out how much of a loser, bad actor, unprofessional, I was.

Suddenly, out of nowhere, a voice sang out.

"Give him his line," George the director said.

The script girl prompted me with a few words of my lines in a monotone that explained the whole experience just by her tone.

Right then and there I knew this thing happens all the time.

She said "Hey, you're the guys that..."

And bam! It all came to back to me. Ego, who was in so much fear of failure and being found out what a fraud. I was making the body light headed with anxiety overload, but was rebooting and back in the saddle. The embarrassment was gone. Ego was in control again. I spewed those lines out and began to act.

Fly:

Self saved the moment, but barely. Ego wanted to quit and run, but self, who is always calm would not let it. That was your conditioning by your father. "Quitters never win and winners never quit". That old Vince Lombardi quote came into your mind.

You blocked and rehearsed one more time and each time, because you knew your lines so well, you where able to act like your character was suppose too. As directed by the director and as the character the Ego saw within the lines. You gained confidence. You felt the part. At this time you went into alpha consciousness, at one with time and space. Everything slows down and it is like the speed is altered at that moment and everything flows like a river: smooth and easy. That's what you felt when you were really acting, being that character for a few seconds. You remember the experience as awesome. Alpha Consciousness is awesome, peaceful, no worries. Now you wanted more. Your Ego grew and self grew with it.

Being an actor was your new mask, justifying the bodybuilding you had been doing for years to protect self, by using Ego to develop muscles, so bullies wouldn't bother you. Now you where an actor. You always wanted to be like Arnold. It enabled your Ego to justify your intense workouts and disciplined lifestyle and acting made money to put food on the table for the kids at the time. Your Ego grew because you fooled them. You were now playing the part of an actor, another mask and role. But it wasn't really true self. It was a role you played, and it was justified by Ego with increased self esteem and great money. But acting was never a passion of yours. It was the possibility of fame and fortune for the Ego. So the Ego was still running the ship. Another piece of your puzzle.

Chapter 8

The Life Puzzle

Mansfield:

What is this puzzle you speak of?

Fly:

Your puzzle is your life picture. Each single experience, each period in your life, everything that you have met, seen, felt, smelled or tasted, is a moment in your time that has been labelled by the Ego as good, bad, or irrelevant to your own life. Each one of these things is a piece to your life puzzle. It is only when you become aware, that these pieces start to fit together to find some clearer picture of who you really are and what realizations about the journey of your life. How all your life experiences up until now have shaped your life. You can pin point on how making certain decisions, at certain times in your life has affected and contributed to the person you are today and how it has shaped your life. Some things could be good, some could be bad, but it gives you a clearer picture of true self.

Once you awake, life becomes fascinating again, as if you where a child learning all over again, but without the insecurity of being emotionally vulnerable, because now at fifty, you have experienced all you dreamed of experiencing growing up. Now you have life experience. So really, no emotion is new anymore. Since your emotions dictate your health and control over emotions creates stability, physically over the body, you are now able to control your own health. You are aware of Ego and because you have experienced all Ego wanted to experience, Ego is bored with the things it has already done. Ego always needs to be entertained, so now Ego and self can work together and do the right thing more frequently and keep health of the body as the number one priority. Being mindful is the key.

Mindfulness of a Fly on the Wall

Chapter 9

What Is Mindfulness?

Practice creates calm

Mansfield: What is Mindfulness, Fly?

Fly:

Mindfulness is the realization of now. Dissuading the Ego, who can only live in your mind in the past and in the future?

Now is the only state the human being is ever physically present in. So, you think now, what you eat now, what you drink now, how you sleep, all have a bearing on tomorrow. But *now* is the key. Nature is now. Now is being in the moment. Bringing yourself back to now and doing it on a regular basis (practice) to become aware and making Ego, self and body together as one is the ultimate goal.

Mansfield:
How can we become more aware?
Fly:
One way is stop complaining! The number one thing is one of the easiest things to become conscious of and stop. We are always in now. A complaint is something about the past and worries about the future that we can't do anything about right now. A complaint is all Ego. All about "Me" ...." he cut me off, he's a bad driver, why do I have to work? etc. Nothing can be done after the fact to deal with now. A complaint generates negative energy that is being sent out into the world. When you complain, cortisol and stress hormones are released into the blood streams that are detrimental to the body's health. When you complain, your Ego is looking for justification on the situation, and is looking for allies. A complaint is wasted energy in the moment.

This exercise will make you more aware. Because every time you complain your Ego is the one that doesn't want self to get hurt again. And once you realize that a complaint only comes from the Ego, you will become more aware and mindful of how much your own conditioning of your Ego and how your Ego came to be.

Mansfield:

Yes, I remember when I was in car sales in 1994. I had just moved from a dealership that was Pontiac Buick—Cadillac, to a Saturn dealership.

An old veteran car salesman named Jack was the top dog. He could sell cars like there was no tomorrow. When he was with a potential buyer, he was in his element. I truly believe that when Jack was in the process of selling a car he was doing what he was born to do. His energy was high. You could see the endorphins racing through his body. His eyes and smile would change. He was truly happy.

Being a car salesman, sometimes, the traffic into the dealership is slow. All the salesmen would gather together to kill time until the next potential customer would arrive on the lot. We would then take turns serving the customers who arrived on the car lot. A *who's up to bat* sort of thing. You had to know your order, or you could get scooped by another salesman, meaning if you weren't there, another salesman could grab your turn. The order was usually determined in order of who arrived first at the dealership in the morning and Jack was always first.

Sometimes it would be a few hours at a time where no one would show up to look at cars. Jack would start to complain. He would complain about management, the weather, the economy, the Toronto Maple Leaf's, the weather again, pretty much everything. He would complain about the people coming onto the lot to look at cars, and find a reason why "They are not buying today".

He would bring everyone down and put them in a bad mood. All the negative energy that was created by the complaints made everyone as angry as Jack. So, when it was your turn to go out and greet a customer and try to present a car, and sell it, the negative energy from all the complaining took me out of the mood to present a car. With all the complaining it made me feel like these people were just looking at cars, were bothering us, were complaining about life. I felt like I needed to get back to the complaining with Jack. I didn't feel like trying to sell a car.

The only thing I noticed was that Jack could flick a switch in his own mind and sell a car no matter how much complaining he did to us. He was an old veteran salesman and could sell a car in his sleep if he wanted to. The only time he could find his contentment, was when he was putting a car deal together.

One thing that struck me as odd at the time, was that the energy he produced from his complaining affected his body. He had heart problems, he was on nitro glycerine. He wasn't a very healthy person.

Why would a guy who can sell a car a day and is well off financially, complain so much?

Fly:

Jack, yes, I remember him well. His negative attitude helped contribute to his heart condition along with his poor diet. He was a sweet, kind hearted man, but his glass was always half empty. I would guess he complained so much because that is the way he was conditioned. He had role models who where complainers. Some people complain, just to start a conversation. A complaint is negative energy given out into the world. Will you accept that negative energy with your receiver and complain some more to empathize with that person who is complaining and justify their Ego? Or will you let it pass and not engage in that conversation? That conversation could actually affect your physical health.

Mansfield:

Are there any other ways to become mindful?

Fly:

Try and realize with every situation or experience, once you are engaged in it, respond, don't react emotionally. Try and leave emotions out of the situation.

Emotions are the gateway to realizing your own health. Control of emotion is control of health. When you can choose which emotions you want to feel and which ones you want to minimize, then you can control your health.

Meditation is the best way to separate your-*self* from Ego. There are many ways to meditate, you will have to find one that suits your way of eliminating the Ego for a while and just *BE*.

A quick way to bring yourself back to now is to watch the wind blow through the trees for twenty seconds. Watch the way the wind moves each branch of leaves. Do they move in unison or do they move separately? Does the wind move all the trees at the same time or just some?

How fast do they move? Does it matter what kind of tree it is? Do all branches of different trees move the same?

This exercise will bring you back to now, while Ego will be in the back of your head yelling;

"This is a stupid waste of time!"

"There are more important things to be doing!"

"What will this accomplish; we have other things to do!"

"We are wasting time."

This is where you begin to train Ego to become the passenger. Ego only cares about the future or past, it hates right now unless it is physically active in an activity that entertains it.

If you can continue to do this exercise, soon Ego goes along with now and realizes that a few seconds to come back to now, keeps all negative emotions in check.

Mansfield;

Why Meditate?

Fly;

Meditation brings the physical brain waves to Alpha consciousness, which is most beneficial to the health of the human body. It is almost as good as delta. Alpha is an awake state, totally focused; all functions of the body are relaxed and functioning. Sometimes repetitive physical work that has been programmed into the psyche through repetition can have someone in a meditative state. In alpha consciousness there is no time.

For example, driving to work, deep in thought about something pleasant, you don't even realize how you drove twenty-three miles to work, unaware of time, body and mind relaxed. You have to come back to beta consciousness to go into work and start to communicate with other humans. And here's Ego, ready to do battle, ready to protect you.

Mansfield:

Why be more aware or mindful?

Fly:

The more mindful you are, the more in tune you are with your body, soul and nature. It becomes a new journey as you become in line with nature and the universe. As you become more aware you start to be able to control your emotions. Eliminate the bad as best as possible and focus on the good positive emotions of love, kindness, peace, gratitude and compassion. Practising Ego awareness will slowly, over time, start to eliminate stress. Becoming more aware benefits the body by not having to deal with all the emotional drama of reactions to experiences that produce all sorts of negative hormones the body has to process. The negative emotions of the Ego, defending itself, somewhere, sometime, a lot of times, only in our own minds. How many wars have you fought in your head with someone you had a misunderstanding with? Lots of worry, stress, lots of what ifs? What does this mean now? etc.

That's Ego worrying. That's what Ego does best. Unfortunately, worry leads to stress and hurts the body.

Becoming more mindful helps you control Ego and will contribute to your own well being.

The more mindful you are the more spiritual you become, because you begin to realize that everything belongs as a whole. There is nothing separate, all nature, man and the creator, God, are all one entity now.

When you are mindful, you spend more time in alpha consciousness and that is a stress-less state.

Once you begin to live your life with this mind set, the possibilities are amazing.

If you where to have the ultimate diet, exercise and spiritual plan, to have mind body and spirit as one, the evolution of the human mind and brain could be taken to another level of consciousness.

As you practise being more aware of your own mind, which is Ego and realize why you want to make a decision before you actually make it, then the road to true self actualization has begun and is going to be ever changing and growing.

Chapter 10

Soul

What is Self Actualization?

Mansfield:

What does self actualization feel like?

Fly:

This is the feeling of total contentment and peace. Realizing who you really are is a moment in time. Your whole life is a blink of an eye in time and you feel it and are content about it. You know and have experienced all emotions and have the choice on which ones are healthy to the body and which ones are not healthy or detrimental to the body. You have experienced all situations that you could ever want to experience and all the ones you didn't want to experience. Now you can avoid situations that would compromise true self and embrace the emotions that are healthy energy to the body and make it heal and feel good. Now you have some control. Control over Ego and the control of your own health, as much as God will allow. If you honor the body, you honor God. God is now. God is love. We are made in God's image, so strive for love, creativity, peace and contentment. Worry free, guilt free, anxiety free is your life now.

The universe is flowing along like a river and you flow along with it. There may be times you come across some shallow water or some rocks that you get snagged on for a short time as there are always rocks and shallow waters in life. But that is life. The key is to be mindful so it doesn't affect your health and respond logically to deal with the situation. You already have the experience in life to break away and continue flowing down that river. When you are young and Ego is still being developed, there are many shallow spots in your river, rocks, even boulders and dead trees sometimes. Now, when you are self actualized the river is clear and wide open. You seem to be able to deal with it all and move on with the least amount of anxiety. Every day is like summer holidays when you were a kid.

Maslow categorised fifteen characteristics that a self-actualized person would realize.

- Perceive reality efficiently and can tolerate uncertainty
- Accept themselves and others for who they are
- Spontaneous in thought and action
- Problem centered and not self centered
- Unusual sense of humor
- Able to look at life objectively
- Highly creative
- Resistant to enculturation, but not purposely unconventional
- Concerned for welfare of humanity
- Capable of deep appreciation of life experiences
- Establish deep satisfying interpersonal relationships with a few people
- Peak experience
- Need for privacy
- Democratic attitude
- Strong moral and ethical standards

Maslow states that once self-actualization is met, all or some of these characteristics may be recognizable for each individual and self-actualization is unique to each individual.

Mansfield:

Where can I read more about Ego, conditioning and awareness?

Fly:

The humorous thing about the manual to live a long healthy life has been right in front of the human race for thousands of years. It is New Testament of the Holy Bible and it tells it like it is. It is a health manual for a long life. Jesus was the teacher of Ego and how to control and relinquish it for the health of the human body. Jesus taught the truth.

The teachings of Jesus show about man's Ego and how it works. Freud figured this out and devised treatments to overcome one's conditioning. Jesus brought it to the people. Freud defined it into a science.

As was stated before, the body is a physical receiver of energies that flow throughout the universe. The better tuned into the positive life-giving energy the physical body is, the healthier the body and mind of the person is.

The teachings of Jesus eliminates stress from the human condition. If one has no stress, the body's systems will function at optimum levels. If nutrition, sleep, exercise, and hydration are optimized, then the evolution of man would take the next step: Mind, body and soul, as one. As Jesus was.

Mansfield:
Where does it say this in the Bible?
Fly;
The New Testament is all about controlling Ego, receiving energy and reaching for that ultimate goal. Mind, body and soul, as one. Heaven on Earth.

Jesus said **"Deny thy self"** which truly means deny your Ego. Get to know the difference between Ego and super Ego (self) so you can control Ego, control emotions, control health. Jesus was teaching mind, body, and soul as one.

Jesus had no Ego. He demonstrated that by washing other people's feet. He did not judge others, he spoke to and taught all walks of life.

Jesus died on the cross, saying, "Forgive them father for they know not what they do."

Timothy 2 13: "If we believe not, yet he abideth faithful: he cannot deny himself."

If we say we believe in Jesus' word, and practise all rituals, but really in our hearts don't believe, then there is no way you can deny Ego. Ego and previous conditioning still exist and controls the mind. Ego will find a way to justify what it wants. Truly what the mind thinks the body will follow.

Mark 1:15: "Repent ye, and believe the gospel". This means, re-think your conditioning or re-think your ways. Your ways are your conditioning.

Matthew 5:5

"Blessed are the meek, for they shall inherit the earth." Meek in those times meant humble. If you are humble, your mind set is as a giver. Giving positive energy out to the universe. While the Ego tends to be selfish and if any love is to be given it will be on Ego's terms.

Luke 17; 21

"Neither shall they say, Lo here or Lo there, the Kingdom of God is within you". You can't point to the Kingdom of God that Jesus talks about. It is within you, when you get over your conditioning and start to work towards becoming Ego free, as Jesus was. Live in the love, energy, healing the body of bad chemicals, cortisol, and stress. These challenges are internal within consciousness. Jesus was a teacher on controlling Ego. Ego and self meld together as one when self actualized. What the mind believes the body will follow.

Old testament example of Ego:

Genesis: For Adam to eat the apple, his Ego decided that he would disobey God. When God confronted Adam, he passed blame to Eve. Adam said: "Wasn't my fault. She gave it to me." Ego got the better of Adam as his thoughts would have been of curiosity of what would happen if he did eat the apple and that who is God to deny me? Curiosity is part of Ego.

1 Corinthians 1-3 "If I do as I should do and I do not have love, I gain nothing".

Humans need love for survival, they need to give it and receive it. It is a cycle, like everything else. The human body feeds on the energy produced when one feels love. Remember we are receivers of energies we can't measure or see. Ego is the one who is self-centred, proud, arrogant and insecure. Acknowledge Ego, acknowledge Jesus. Learn and move on. Be conscious of living in Love. It is way easier and less stressful. Love is a positive energy we need for our own survival.

If you don't have love, your physical body starts to deteriorate.

We are products of love and need to give love in order for all receiving of love to be successfully accepted by the body.

Pride and arrogance are bad emotions for the body to exude. They block love trying to feed the body and the body starves if it doesn't receive enough love energy.

To be too proud or arrogant to give love, or to be too insecure to give love, robs the receptors in the body from getting any back. The energy is blocked.

Chapter 11

God and the Devil

Mansfield:
What are God and the Devil?

Fly:
Bringing everything full circle from the beginning of when humans first appeared on this planet is still up for debate. It is all speculation on our existence.

God, for what this Fly has seen, is simply now. There is a flow of the universe that continues every moment and as a consciousness we have to bring ourselves back to the moment to find any peace within ourselves. There is all the energy, that if you practice unconditional love without judgements, without boundaries, not wanting, then the energies we attract will be positive and that will be physically positive for the health of the body. What the mind believes the body will follow.

Believe in God and let God's will be done. You are just here to respond to what comes at you unemotionally, or pick what emotion and how much you want to show. Then stress will begin to dissipate within your life. That's what the ten commandments are for. The health of the body. With the correct discipline, integrity, and preparation to purpose, you will know God better and leave Ego as a distant voice.

As for that Devil, he was created to destroy you. He was always the manifestation of negative energy produced by Ego and the mind living in the past and dreaming of a future of pleasure. Ego is the one who wants to take control. If you substitute Ego for Devil, or Satan, etc. in the Holy Bible, it might make more sense for some. This is what Jesus was teaching.

The Devil and Ego go hand and hand. Ego, or "I", is being selfish, keeping your love from others and not receiving any because you are too closed minded and have built a wall between.

Being selfish immediately brings you to thinking about how your future will look or be perceived with thinking about "I". It's all about me; everyone for himself. That is the Devil and negative energy receiver. Ego physically hurts the body with stress hormones. Jesus' teaching shows how to control Ego through discipline of one's thoughts and actions. The Bible shows that throughout its pages, but be aware, it was written by men who had Egos too.

Chapter 12

Discipline of Mind

Mansfield:

How can we physically help change our consciousness?

Fly:

Exercise! The human body is meant to move. Exercise brings you back to *now*, back to the moment. This is why Ego hates to exercise if it isn't in your conditioning. It is imperative that you keep your vessel or receiver of energy at a high level of fitness. The more fit you are, the better your body receives positive energy from others and the universe, healing your body from the day's endeavours. Your body is like a tuning fork, Sensitive to energy and flow. Keep it tuned and become part of the universe. Become able to control Ego with the ultimate goal of mind, body and soul, as one.

Your body is a gift, given to you as your means of getting around in this formed world. It grows and changes with time. It is remarkable how the human body can heal itself from disease, tears, breaks, etc. It is the most valuable machine you will ever use. Yet a lot of you do not take care of it. It is a last priority for some.

You Say "Life is too busy, I don't have time to exercise." (Ego is full of excuses.)

This is not what God intended the body for. Doctors say you need to exercise to be healthy, but they know full well that the Ego will compromise on that subject. Hard work goes against the Ego because exercising makes you stay in the moment. Ego only lives in the past or future. If it is in the now, then it needs to be entertained. It is too hard to stay in the moment and concentrate only on what you are doing and it might be uncomfortable physically. Ego hates discomfort, even if it will benefit your overall health.

1 Corinthians 6, 19-20 "What? Know ye not that your body is the temple of the Holy Ghost which is in you which ye have of God and ye are not your own. For ye are bought with a price: therefore, glorify god in your body and in your spirit, which are gods. The Holy Spirit lives within the body: Honor thy body."

When you honor your body, you honor God for this gift he has bestowed to you.

Isaiah 40 28-31 "Do not let yourself get weary."

Take care of yourself, eat when you are supposed to eat, sleep when you are supposed to sleep, exercise when you are supposed to exercise. You can't give love if you are sick. You have to take care of yourself. Fatigue makes cowards of us all. With fatigue comes sickness which awakens Ego. You will know it when the first complaint pops into your head.

Romans 12, 1

"...that ye present your body as living sacrifice, holy, acceptable unto God, which is your reasonable service."

This means that you must take care of the body and it will be difficult. You must live in sacrifice (meaning eat right, sleep right, exercise right) to make sure you are healthy enough to worship God. If you live in sacrifice, this means to live a balanced life. Sometimes you have to sacrifice eating certain foods that are detrimental to the health of the body and you have to sacrifice time at the gym, to take care of the vessel. Life is always sacrifice, even though the Ego will convince self that it doesn't have to sacrifice. Ego wants a piece of cake and eat it too.

Mansfield:

Sacrifice huh? What are the best ways to train your mind and body as one? How will I look at life now that I know you, the Fly, are here?

Fly:

Now that you are aware, you can never go back to living unconsciously through Ego, for it is a lie to self and self needs truth always.

That's why Jesus said "I am the way. I am the truth."

He endorsed the Ten Commandments because they teach discipline. Discipline creates energy that is beneficial to the vessel.

Exodus 20 3-17

Ten Commandments

- ONE: Thou shall be no other gods before me. Worship now, God is now, god is love energy. Be grateful that you are still here and alive. Are you worshipping money and don't realize it?

Keep Ego focused on worship of God. The Ego and mind need to stay focused on a goal. We are purely spiritual beings, giving and receiving energy. Worship can bring Ego and self together to attain one goal and that is to above all else, worship god. This creates a stress-free life, physically for the body and mentally for self and Ego. To give up control, which is the goal of the Ego, is to control each situation so as not to let true self be found out or hurt. When you start to lose Ego and self emerges, it then comes down to "God willing".

- TWO: No false gods or idolatry. No image made to be worshipped. Discipline

  Ego needs something to focus on. You can't worship God and money at the same time.

  Many don't even realize they are practising idolatry when they are worshipping money. Jesus would ask followers to drop your wealth now and follow the word of God. Not many did. Their own Ego's would not let them.

- THREE: Thou shall not take the Lord's name in vain.

Discipline

This commandment would be direct training on disciplining the Ego not to swear or curse. This creates negative energy expelled from the body. And the way it works is: "What you put out, you receive twice as much back."

- FOUR Remember the Sabbath day.

More **discipline** training for the body to rest from work so body can heal and create some spiritual time. The Sabbath day is a time to reflect on the past week and live in gratitude for what you have. It is the time to reflect on how you gave of yourself to others during the week. This is training Ego, for mind, body and soul connection.

- FIVE: Honor thy father and mother.

Honor your conditioning. Everything happens as God's will. Everything happens for a reason. Whatever your circumstance, honor your conditioning, realize what it is, good or bad and move on and focus on God. God is the moment. Keep Ego focused on God, not what you have or haven't got, or what was done to you, or why? Realize Ego always has to have a purpose, a goal, or something to concentrate on. Health wise, God is the only answer. God is physically good for the body.

Accepting "It is what it is". I am here now, so move on.

- SIX: Thou shall not kill.
- You have to control Ego not to kill, but social consciousness of groups can make Ego justify killing, such as war over injustice or land, or money. Anyone that kills, deals with negative energy for the rest of their lives. This negative energy will be a scar that never heals. This is the most negative energy ever for the body to handle. It never leaves you and will always be with you. It creates a negative energy receiver, feeling all negative emotions at once, all the time.
- SEVEN: Thou shall not commit adultery.

Brings Ego all sorts of negative energy emotions. What Ego wants, Ego gets. Ego will always justify everything it does. It will leave the body with tons of cortisol. Adultery brings on all of the negative emotions. Jealousy, guilt, lust, control, power and worry, all filled and associated with more stress. STD's destroy the body from the inside out.

- EIGHT: Thou shall not steal.
  Ego working on negative emotions again…plus, not wanting to get caught. Paranoia, anxiety, worry, fear, are all detrimental to the health of the body.
- NINE: Thou shall not bear false witness against thy neighbor.
  Don't lie. When you do you create stress. One lie leads to another lie and Ego needs to cover its tracks producing guilty, worry, dishonesty, etc.
- TEN: Thou shall not covet.
  Be happy with what you have. If you worship God and have true, faith and contentment, peace start to enter your life, stress begins to dissipate and Ego cannot live in the present moment. God is and always is "Now". Wanting is a product of the Ego.

As Jesus endorsed Gods rules for man, he is basically guiding the consciousness of man and showing how he should live to lead a long and happy life. If you follow these ten basic rules in a human's life the energy that you attract will be more positive, you have way less stress and the body can deal with all the negative, naturally produced chemicals.

Remember exercise, diet, sleep, and proper hydrations are also required. These are required to honor God and all this discipline trains you to be conscious *now*.

Fly: Analyse the Seven Deadly Sins from the book, *Dante's Inferno*: lust, gluttony, greed, sloth, wrath, envy, and pride. The lesson here is about negative emotions which will produce negative chemicals within the body, changing the PH levels to a disease endorsing environment. These sins will destroy the body from inside out. This is what Jesus tried to convey all those years ago. Negative emotions bring negative detrimental chemicals to the body. All these negative emotions bring worry, strife, guilt and resentment to the body.

Lust: 2 Timothy 2:22 "Flee also youthful lust; but pursue righteousness, faith, love, and peace"...Chastity and self control cures lust by controlling passion and leverages energy for the good of others.

Gluttony: 1 Corinthians 10:31 "Therefore, whether you eat or drink, or whatever you do, do all to the glory of God."

Temperance cures gluttony by implanting the desire to be healthy, therefore making one fit to serve others.

Greed: 1Timothy 6:10 "For the love of money is the root of all evil: while some coveted after, they have erred from faith, and pierced themselves through and with many sorrows."

Sloth: 2 Thessalonians 3:10 "For even when we were you, this we command you, that if any would not work neither should they eat."

Wrath: Romans 12:19 "Beloved, never avenge yourself, but leave it to the wrath of God, for it is written, vengeance is mine, I will repay says the Lord."

Envy: Proverbs 14:30 "A sound heart is life to the body, but envy is rottenness to the bones."

Pride: Proverbs 16:18 "Pride goethe before destruction, and haughty spirit before a fall."

Chapter 13

Energy of Life

Mansfield:

What is this energy you talk about, which the body receives?

Fly:

First of all, we must look at human biology. Science has proven that the body is fueled by electrical impulses from the brain to the body in order to function. When a person has a heart attack, they are revived by an electrical current that re-starts the heart and the goal would be to get a normal heart rhythm. So logically it makes sense that the human body receives and gives off, uses and distributes energy.

The energy that flows throughout the universe is endless. We can only feel about 5% of what is in the universe in terms of energy, but we are living with 95% of the universe's energy that we never see, feel, taste, touch or smell. The energy that humans receive and give off is positive and negative ions and are felt with our emotional conditioning.

Positive ions are created with approaching thunderstorms, electronic devices, negative emotions and feelings. These are all electrical currents that the body responds negatively to. Negative energy is felt in our negative emotions. When we are angry, upset, jealous, guilty, worried, etc., these give off negative energy.

Negative ions are good and beneficial to the body. They are created by nature, waterfalls, trees and plants and positive human emotion. (Love)

When healthy children are young, toddler age, they are finely tuned instruments receiving energy with no Egoic baggage, no pre-determined Egoic future or past. They are just receivers of energy. The energy they get from the parents' love is all they know, positive and negative, sensitive to both.

How many times have you ever noticed a burst of energy from a toddler? It is like something passed through them and they explode with joy. Then they become calm again. It had nothing to do with what they ate or drank; it was just a burst of energy. A burst of joy or happiness.

You can remember that feeling, can't you? You can remember it now, just recently, because you are beginning to get those bursts of energy again as an adult. BOH, or burst of happiness, is what you have been calling them. BOH's are positive energy flowing through the universe at the time and you just happen to be in their path. They flow right through you, heal you, let you know that all is being taken care of by the Lord and you have no worries. They come when the body is in peak physical condition, which now is always, because you have learned, practised and lived what is now.

BOH's have always and will always flow throughout the universe, but as humans get older they stop the exercising, they stop moving, they get lazy. They eat wrong and get no sleep, so their receivers (bodies) break down. They get lost in Ego, because Ego is lazy and doesn't want to do anything more than it has too. They are unconscious and ignorant and don't want to change because deep down their self is afraid and they only know their conditioning.

Negative ions are in high quantity after a thunderstorm. This is when you should open your windows and let the air blow throughout the house. These negative ions leave the body calm and relaxed. Your brain waves are closer to alpha consciousness. With practise you can live in alpha consciousness almost all the time.

When you choose to react emotionally to a situation where negative energy from negative emotions are directed your way, you physically accept that energy and react emotionally. Huge amounts of negative chemicals are dumped into the blood stream. They create a poisonous acidic environment for disease to grow. The more you are unaware of your reactions, the more you condition your body and mind to attract that very same negative energy and the ultimate outcome, as Jesus states, will be death.

Respond knowing the negative energy is there, but choose not to accept the energy internally and respond accordingly, controlling the physical state of the body and mind. The negative hormones released from the body will be only small, if any, with good practise. You need to be aware when it is the negative energy and choose to deal with it as quickly as possible, to eliminate the worry associated with that negative energy.

Chapter 14

States of Consciousness

Mansfield:

What happens in alpha consciousness?

Fly:

Calm. Peace. Quiet. Ego is sleeping when you are in alpha. This is where self can be self. It is in your own head. There is no time when in alpha. To be in alpha consciousness always, would mean the elimination of Ego vs. self. They have become one. Responding to everything. Not reacting emotionally. Constant control of your emotions, letting your emotions come to you and deciding which ones are beneficial to the body and which ones are not.

This also benefits the body physically, because you would be in a constant healing state for the body. Maybe new things would be activated in the brain because you only use ten percent of the capacity. Your Ego has been created and received its' training in beta consciousness and only has control of what you do in beta until you realize your conditioning and why you do and feel the way you do in certain situations.

Mansfield:

What is Beta Consciousness?

Fly:

This is where your Ego was created and dwells. Like a monster in a movie, from day one, your Ego was conditioned. Conditioned to eat, sleep, talk, walk, dress, act, everything we live every day is beta consciousness. Everything labelled by logic is Ego. Beta conscious is how you communicate with each other, as humans. Your thoughts are most often motivated by Ego before you speak them, but you have to come to beta consciousness in order to communicate them to the world. All human communication that we have labelled, so far, can be defined as beta consciousness.

Example: We can be in alpha, daydreaming and someone comes up and starts a conversation. Now we have to come back to beta to concentrate and communicate with that person and listen in beta consciousness and answer in beta . Beta is the world we live in. We have to be in beta to comprehend what is going on around us, with a label for everything. This is where Ego creates your stress.

We live in a material world of physical properties. In other worlds, we need to feed and clothe ourselves. We need shelter. If you could condition yourself to do your job, while still being able to slip in and out of beta/alpha at will, anew consciousness could be formed and you would have ultimate health for mind, body and soul.

Self is in alpha and has to be heard in beta, but is first filtered by Ego with labels, knowledge and time, before expressed.

Mansfield:

Is there anything that can help my meditation to get to alpha consciousness quicker?

Fly:

Marijuana can transform your consciousness from beta to alpha. Basically, when you inhale marijuana your consciousness begins to change. You start to drift away from beta consciousness, where Ego is in charge, which are thoughts of the past or future. You start to view the world in a different way, through alpha consciousness. It is your own personal view of you with no Ego. This transition from beta to alpha can scare people because their Ego does not want to let go and be pushed away. This can bring anxiety during the transition of consciousness, but it soon passes. As the body ascends to alpha, it starts to release the negative energy held tight within the body. You can physically feel this.

The nerve endings awaken and you are more aware of your surroundings. You can actually sit one moment and have no thoughts at all then be deep in thought the next. In alpha your Ego isn't there anymore. That is why it is used in meditation. It can be a tool to relax and change consciousness; to be able to just be one with now, with nature and the universe. It heals the body, relaxes the mind, and feeds the soul.

Mansfield:

Sounds awesome, but I have to work. My job is stressful. I need to make money to survive.

Fly:

Everyone has to work to pay their own way, but how and what they do is different for each individual. They are again, products of their own conditioning.

Ask yourself if you absolutely love your job, or are you there only because of the money, power, esteem etc.? Are you at peace with yourself? Are you content? Do you love your life? Or is it a constant war being fought every day within your own mind? Can you relax?

The money at whatever job should always be a means to an end to be able to follow your passion and pursue mind, body and soul, as one.

Mansfield:

What if I don't have a passion or haven't found it yet?

Fly:

If you don't have a passion, meaning an activity you just love to do, even if it has nothing to do with making money, ask yourself if you might be too absorbed with making money, or too self absorbed. You could be worshipping money over God. You could be "lost in Ego", as a lot of people are.

Lost in Ego means that all your daily activities are so labelled and categorized by your Ego that it becomes draining, unexciting, stressful and anxious. It will never be fun because there is no end. Ego will never be satisfied.

If you work toward getting your vessel in absolutely the best physical shape, place your spirit on Jesus and your mind on being mindful of Ego and true self, you will change and you will find a passion for something.

Make health your number one priority: mind, body and soul, as one. A new you will emerge. But be mindful that there is no money in it. Just optimum health, joy and contentment. You can find peace here once that is achieved. Be aware that once you find your passion, if you decide to turn your passion into a way of making money, it may become its own burden, rather than continue to be your passion. Money should be a means to an end for your passion.

Chapter 15

Re-Conditioning Yourself

Mansfield:

What is my state of mind when I re-condition myself?

Fly:

There are three states of thinking when consciously trying to re-conditioning one's mind. It will take a while because of old conditioning habits. You have to begin trying to be conscious of three states of mind, when performing your daily tasks. Categorise these in the following three states of mind: (Eckert Tolle)

You live in acceptance of what you have to do. This is your work, job, or career. Is your job acceptable for the health of your body? Is it low stress and enough pay to continue to follow your passions? Can you continue to do this activity with some type of enjoyment and continue to pay your way in the world while leaving low stress levels to the body? This is acceptance.

You live in excitement of what you get to do. This is quitting time and your time. Free time to do whatever you want. Your Ego is always a little more energetic around quitting time because it releases adrenaline and endorphins which make you feel awake, alert and strong. Ego likes quitting time.

Example 1: One day you might have nothing planned after work, but you are still joyful when it is time to go home and just relax. The Ego sees the light at the end of the tunnel on this specific day. Ego always associates things with time. You still are excited even though nothing new is going on.

Example 2: If you had big plans like a ticket to a show you want to see. The anticipation and excitement are at a higher level on this day. Both days you have the excitement, but some days have more excitement than others.

Enthusiasm is in what you love as your passion or the thing that gives you most joy when you are doing it. When you are participating in your passion, and you could have more than one, you will find that time doesn't exist, it just flies by. Only you, the individual, will know what your true passion is. These passions are where you will find your ability to flow into alpha consciousness, be creative within your passion, and keep discovering new passions.

If you live in these three states of mind, you will have control over your emotions. If you have control over your emotions, you become closer to your true self and nature. Self emerges with the education of all that Ego has learned and Ego is now the background player in your puzzle. Always there, but just a faint voice, ready to help from previous experiences if needed.

If you have control over your emotions and your Ego, you will have control over your own health.

Mansfield:

Yeah sure, easy for you to say, but how do I accomplish that?

Fly:

First you have to remember to always have in your mind Acceptance, Excitement, Enthusiasm.

Then add these words to your new life puzzle because now your picture is starting to take shape. You have to practice being now with these mindful exercises. It will take great discipline.

Chapter 16

Live in Excellence

"Perfection is not attainable, but with the pursuit of perfection brings excellence." *Vince Lombardi.*

<u>D.I.P.</u>
Discipline
Integrity
Preparation

Discipline: Discipline your day with what you need to accomplish for that day. You are only concerned with today and nothing else. Your focus is only on today, not on what is happening tomorrow or sometime in the future. You have to discipline yourself to be in this moment. You have to discipline yourself to exercise every day, eat right, and go to bed at the required time for full healing. You have to discipline your Ego by following those Ten Commandments that Jesus talked about. You need to discipline yourself to follow how you conduct yourself amongst others. You need to discipline yourself to be prepared and live with integrity. This is what the human body needs for good health and peace of mind. Discipline is what controls Ego and sets humans apart from the animals. Without discipline life is unfulfilling.

"The Good Lord gave you a body that can withstand anything; it is the mind you have to convince." *Vince Lombardi.*

Integrity

Integrity is a large category to bring to the table. It is, basically, your truth. Integrity is doing your job 110% everyday. Even if you don't like your job, you must continue to do your absolute best and have a good attitude about it. Integrity is honesty. Integrity is being on time and integrity is spreading love and positive energy daily. It is helping. It is doing what you say, saying what you do. Integrity is not complaining, not gossiping, not knowingly or purposely trying to hurt someone emotionally or physically. Integrity is not leaving a foot print where you have been so no one has to clean up after you. It is when you pick an item up in the grocery store and decide when you are at the cash register you don't want it anymore and you take it back to the exact shelf you picked it from. That's integrity. When you help someone and do something out of love and you don't go around boasting about how good a person you are, that is integrity. You should be same person alone, as when you are around others.

Preparation: You have to be prepared for whatever task awaits you. From having to have a report done on time, studying for a test, preparing one's food for the day or memorizing lines for tomorrow's shoot. These all have to be prepared for. This will then eliminate stress and recondition the body to adapt to the life style. Repetitive preparation of one's day will eventually become a way of life and therefore lower cortisol or stress levels.

If you live with D.I.P. ingrained in your psyche and live a consciousness of acceptance, excitement, and enthusiasm, then you will be "Living in Excellence", as Jesus taught.

Mansfield:

I guess when you look at it truthfully, the Ten Commandments are what discipline and integrity is.

Fly:

Yes, you are correct. They are a guide to self actualization. Mind, body and soul, as one with nature, the universe, and God.

Chapter 17

What is Our Purpose

Mansfield:

What is our true purpose?

Fly:

A human's true purpose is to love and be loved. It is the instinctual need that separates us from the animals we are here to care for. The human needs love to survive. The human body needs love to function properly. Without love, humans have nothing. Human instinct understands it has to love. It is what to love that has become the difficult task. Some people love things that can't love them back and that is a recipe for bad health and eventual death.

Love is a physical energy that exists throughout the universe that humans give and receive. If their receivers, their bodies, are functioning properly, the flow of positive energy benefits the body.

How you love is based on how your own teaching of love was taught to you. Through role models, media, parents, etc., (this is your conditioning). Your true purpose is to love and you need to get over your earlier teaching or conditioning before you can truly love, the way Jesus taught. This is the way the mind, body and soul connection exist with nature.

Mansfield:

What is love?

Fly:

Love is always a choice!

Love is the most important word in the world's language, whatever language you say it in, it means the same. God is love.

Genesis: "Man is made in the image of God."

The human being is programmed to love. To give love away. The human being cannot exist without love. It needs to emit love and receive love regularly in order to exist. If love is withheld indefinitely, it will die of loneliness. Loneliness will manifest itself into stress, worry and eventually the mind will develop physical ailments from all the negative emotion of loneliness and eventually result in physical death.

As Jesus stated in 1 Corinthians 13 1-3: "but if I do not have love, I gain nothing."

All humans love. It is just what they love, where they can go wrong. Or, why they love? Who? How? Etc.

All these complex questions need to be answered by your friend Ego. Humans need to know.

From birth to twenty-five years-old, Ego is being conditioned and brain development is still evolving. Self and Ego are all developing at the same time and whatever is conditioned into the mind on what is love to them, is filtered by the Ego who then labels it. If someone has had a bad experience in love, then that baggage can go with them until, if ever, they realize their conditioning and get over it and move on.

Getting back to love is a choice. We can choose who we want to love. We choose the way we want to love that person. Ego decides who, why, when, how long... what's in it for us? All these good things for self.

Self just wants to love, as it is supposed to do. Ego puts limitations on everything. Ego protects self from getting hurt, emotionally. Ego can sometimes be self destructive because it loses control over self, and tries to compensate by acting in an uncharacteristic way. (acting out of your normal character).

Previous conditioning and experiences play a role in developing love. Love is always developing and changing once Ego is realized and the consciousness of the love switches into alpha consciousness from beta consciousness.

Beta Consciousness Love is rules and regulations on how to love, who to love, how you have sex, when etc. There are lots of words attached to this kind of love...performance is a good word. Alpha Consciousness is love...unconditional. This a feeling, no words can describe.

The love that is developed between a mother and baby is alpha consciousness love. It will never die. It can be buried, deep behind Ego and its rules, but alpha love will never die. It is unconditional.

When you grew up and Ego was being developed, you learned and knew instinctively that you were drawn to love. You were drawn to want to give your love and be loved by others: Friends, girlfriends, family, activities. These are all different kinds of love. The thing is, they are all similar but different. If self wants to give unconditional love all the time and Ego puts limits on who you love, how, why? etc., then giving and receiving love can become difficult, stressful, and hard to manage emotionally. Remember humans are receivers of the energy that runs through the universe. We feel these energies within our emotional states.

Mansfield:

What happens when you think you love someone romantically and love is not returned?

Fly: This hurts Ego deeply. Early on in life, what the adolescent mind thinks of love is gathered from what they have witnessed. They try to mimic and copy everything about what they have seen, heard, felt, etc. Ego believes that the world is over when it is rejected. They will never love again, they just want to die, and then have to deal with these feelings of rejection. Ego hates rejection. It may get to the point of going the complete opposite way and associating that feeling of rejection with the rejecter. An emotional scar that the Ego will remember and make sure you don't feel that rejection ever again in life. The Ego builds walls around love. The Ego can transform love and make the love you give and receive have rules, regulations, limitations and protocols, depending on the scars you receive while being conditioned or trained in life. Humans need love to survive.

Mansfield:

Then that means everyone needs love and love is controlled by Ego while conditioning is taking place.

Fly:

Yes, you got it. Everyone's story is different for how they perceive love to be. As you realize your conditioning and move toward Ego and self melding together, you will start to notice more of the true self emerging; the unconditional love that Jesus speaks of. There are less and less of your rules and regulations on loving and receiving love, but Ego is always there, just isn't as devastating when a rule is broken. Hurt feelings are all Ego.

People have to learn how to love without Ego being involved. Jesus was teaching this while everyone was living love through Ego. Living love through Ego is physically detrimental to the health of the body. It becomes counter-productive to healing itself.

It is like love and its Egoic rules have certain patterns. Once you realize your own patterns then you can realize your conditioning and learn to love like Jesus taught.

The way romantic love begins when you decide you are attracted physically to someone, your Ego makes the rules. The most of the time your choices weren't based on friendship and true love, but on physical attraction and desires of the flesh, as the Bible says.

When you love this way, Ego is in charge. Especially when a relationship is new, Ego is looking for red flags. Red flags are devised by the Ego so self won't be emotionally hurt. This is a game of what is acceptable and what isn't, within what you judge that love interest's character to be.

Ego decided what it will put up with to make things work and what it won't put up with. All-in-all, a brick wall starts to build within the relationship and Ego is always trying to manipulate and change the circumstance to its favour. Sooner or later, the wall that has been built with small bricks of negative experiences against the Ego, is so big, that when the last brick goes into that wall, you can't even see your partner anymore. The relationship usually ends at that point and Ego goes out looking for someone else to give love to, with all the same rules and regulations as before. Once you become aware, the true meaning of real love comes to the surface and self emerges.

When you were young you instinctively knew about how the mind and body needed love, but were conditioned, as we all are, to love through Ego.

Mansfield:

Young love had so many conditions attached to it. All created by Ego and conditioning.

Fly:

All your new emotions with girls came up at a younger age than most. You had a serious older girlfriend in Grade Eight: Thirteen years-old, lots of negative emotions because of insecurity, jealousy, anger, emotional outburst of destructive energy, all new to Ego.

After that first serious relationship ended and the next one started, each time the Ego would change rules, change the way the walls were built, some faster than others, some slower. Love was always a quest throughout life. Just understanding it was so hard for you. The walls got built no matter what, as long as Ego was involved. In that time, up until age forty-six, all the love that was given or received had all these rule, regulations, walls etc., until you started to awaken and realized yes you need to love and receive love, but learned that if you concentrated on just the giving part of loving, the receiving part came naturally and came back two fold.

Ego steps into the background once your true self has emerged without fear. Love becomes easy. Stress lowers. Inner peace appears in your life.

Loving within Ego is limited because Ego can only live in the past or future. Ego can't love now. There is always a hidden agenda for the future or what was done in the past when love is filtered through Ego.

Unconditional love has no walls, time, future or past. It is now and it is good energy for the body. It is what humans are designed to do. It is a consciousness. Love is God, right now.

Chapter 18

Body

Physical Fitness,

Time to Awaken Your Vessel

Mansfield:

Why get in shape?

Fly:

The body is a biological vessel for your consciousness to drive. It is very similar to playing a video game. Everything affects everything else within the body. The five key things that affect the body are drink, eat, sleep, exercise, and what you think.

When you break it down your body is a biological machine. A machine that man has studied and copied to make his own machines that make life simpler.

If you really think about it, the human body is amazing in its adaptabilities. The way you can increase the work load and the body builds muscle. Sit on the couch all the time, and the body atrophies.

The body needs to move, use the core muscles, sweat to get rid of toxins and breath hard to get blood flowing, every day. That is what is needed for the body to do its' true job and receive energy from the universe.

Every machine needs to be used for what they are made for. You wouldn't drive Formula One race car forty kilometres per hour just to the corner store every day because that is not what it is made for. Non-use will soon make the machine fail. This is the same for your body. It is meant to move, sweat, perform, and be active. This is what it is built to do from the beginnings of man. He hunted and gathered food all day. He slept well at night because of all the daily physical activity. Early man had the prototype for the first machines; his own body!

If your equipment is faulty, (your body) you can't give and receive energy which is required for survival. They say we only see, hear, smell, taste, and feel 5% of what is really in the universe. It only makes sense that we can receive other energies without consciously knowing it, but humans feel it in their emotions.

Mansfield:

What happens if you are negligent in one or more factors of your health of the body?

Fly:

Those five areas mentioned above affect the body on every level. If one area is out of sync, then the others can get pushed out of their own tolerances and health can suffer.

For instance, if you are not getting enough sleep, it can affect your hormones to the point of not being able to assimilate foods properly. This means that your body is storing fats instead of shedding them. This leads to obesity and health problems.

Not enough fluid can lead to headaches, stress, dehydration and fainting. Constant dehydration can lead to more serious health problems.

Not enough exercise slows metabolism down and with no exercise, it's down to a crawl. So that piece of cake you wanted goes straight to fat storage. You sure don't need those extra calories from sitting on your office chair all day. This is contributing to obesity once again.

What you think, is the most important of the five areas for the health of the body. What the mind believes, the body will follow.

Stress creates health problems within the body. Worry, anxiety and thinking about a problem you can't do anything about at that moment are all things that affect the body. If there is no way for the stress hormones and wastes to leave the body, the body becomes toxic and can manifest itself into disease.

Mansfield:

What shouldn't I eat?

Fly:

Diet is the major health issue of our time. We are so caught up in ourselves and our lives that we seek pleasure and life from food.

Anything from fast food to easy pop in the microwave entrees that taste similar to the real thing but aren't. There are countless cooking shows on television now conditioning us to eat that way. The ingredients they put in these foods are the unhealthiest to go into the human body.

We are killing ourselves a slow pharmaceutical death with sugar. Scientists know it, but there is way too much money involved to try to stop it. You have to be self-educated these days.

They teach you in school what they need to teach you, so you will be a good customer to the pharmaceutical companies for your entire life. Most parents are too busy to try and care. They were taught the same way. Most parents of kids still in school are on at least one or two pharmaceuticals a day and some even more. The health issue starts with diet.

Mansfield:

What should I eat?

Fly:

Any food God created (before Ego got a hold of it and said "I can make it better", is easily, efficiently and perfectly assimilated by the body. (If all other factors are in control: sleep, exercise, hydration, and mind.)

To have the body run most efficiently, the body should have a mostly plant-based diet, with only ten to fifteen percent animal protein ratio. So, a 10-70-20. Ten percent protein, seventy percent plant-based carbohydrates, twenty percent fats. Having the fats as eighty percent mono-saturated fats. These ratios would all depend on the activity level of the individual.

Example: A weightlifter's protein and carbohydrate requirements would be different from a long-distance runner due to their different activity levels.

Mansfield:

So, what is your body for?

Fly:

The body, like a machine, when functioning at optimum, can heal itself almost ninety percent of the time when it comes to sickness, skeletal injuries, and disease. The big question is how do we get it there? What would that hold for the real evolution of our brains and bodies, let alone what impact that might have on the actual physical evolution of what the human brain can actually accomplish.

The human body is a receptor for energies that travel throughout the atmosphere and whether we like it or not we are receiving these energies that travel in and throughout our body every minute of every day. The better the heath is in a human the more easily the energies pass through them.

These energies are both positive and negative to the health of the human body. We relay these energies to the brain and we convert them to what our brains understand as emotions. Emotions as we know them are both good and bad and always defined by Ego. Both can produce endorphins, which in turn helps the body, along with adrenaline and cortisol.

The good emotions such as love, compassion, peace, kindness, gratitude and joy, make the body heal itself and feel good. The endorphins race throughout the body and a sense of calm floods the mind. These emotions are beneficial to the body and are needed for survival.

The negative emotions generated by the mind when receiving these energies daily, effect the body in such a negative way that they can linger for a long period of time throughout the body, as these negative energies are reviewed by the Ego over and over again. Creating the experience repetitively and creating the negative reactions in the body, huge amounts of cortisol "the stress hormone" get dumped into the blood stream every time the tape of the unpleasant experience is played in the mind.

One of the keys to good health is being able to control your levels of cortisol.

In a good experience, such as love, kindness or compassion, large amounts of dopamine and endorphins are released, some adrenaline and depending on the situation, cortisol. Based on it being a pleasurable experience, the cortisol levels are a lot lower to nil. This situation is good for the overall health of the body.

In a bad experience such as jealousy, anger, hate, etc., cortisol, along with adrenaline and only some endorphin, are released by the body. It is hard for the body to assimilate all the cortisol that is flowing throughout it. It makes it harder for the body to deal with the other things in life such as diet, exercise, sleep, and hydration. With all the cortisol running through the body, it can't do its job efficiently and health suffers.

The wonderful gift of life that God has given us is the body that we have. It is a magnificent machine that has tried to be duplicated in every way since the beginning of time.

DaVinci studied the human body and made machines. He invented many things based on his study of the human anatomy. Every machine ever made is based on the original study of the human body.

It makes sense then to use machines as an analogy when describing the process in which the mind/body connection is described. The mind body connection is basis of our true nature and our true evolution.

The nervous system is the adapter of the body. It adapts and changes as the environment, food, shelter, and activity change. Body temperatures, sleep habits, food consumption, exercise are changing throughout our lives as we age. We notice as we grow old our bodies change and start to deteriorate.

Mansfield:

Why does the body always adapt?

Fly;

The nervous system tries to adapt to all stimuli for survival. Whether good or bad, over a consistent amount of time, the nervous system will try to adapt as best it can until it can't anymore.

This is why we see some people live to the age of one hundred and some are gone by fifty. It all has to do with the adaptation of the lifestyle of the body and mind. Does the body get time for healing from the experiences it deals with each day? The nervous system will enable the body to adapt over time to handle the work load.

Example: After the first snow fall you shovel the snow and the next day your muscles get sore. By the end of winter you don't get as sore shoveling the snow. Your muscles, or nervous system, has adapted to the work load by adding just enough muscle in the right places, to now handle that new workload.

The nervous system adapts to internal stimuli also. Negative and positive energies that flow, diet, exercise, sleep patterns, etc.; in other words, lifestyle. If one of these things is off, if your cortisol levels are too high, if you're not getting enough sleep for your lifestyle or if diet is bad, the nervous system will try to adapt the best it can. This might not be favourable for long term and short-term health.

This could be why we have an obesity problem in North America, a high rate of mental illness and suicide. Our nervous systems are trying to adapt to our lifestyles, but it is impossible because it does not have the right tools to do the job. It is like working on an engine of a car and not having the correct tools.

Chapter 19

The Neuro Gravity Resistance Lifestyle

<u>*Neuro Gravity Resistance Training.*</u>

Definition; To train the nervous system with specific energy-transferring exercises, creating new neuro pathways to the core and to awaken consciousness of mind to muscle connection.

What Is Neuro Gravity Resistance training? This system of weight training combines traditional weight training with yoga, Tai Chi and cardio mixed together. It is defined as body sculpting.

Objective: By training the nervous system to adapt to the work load by using weights and varying angles of gravity to create new neuro links and create more awareness between mind, body and soul.

Mansfield:

How do you do this? I know how to weight train. What's so different about this weight training?

Fly:

The major difference with this kind of weight training is consciousness. While performing any exercise when practising Neuro Gravity resistance training, what matters is the speed of contraction of the muscle, along with flawless posture.

Flawless posture enables the neuro pathways to travel in a straight line throughout the body. When one's posture is compromised, neuro connections get shut off at the break in posture. The core can't fire each muscle consecutively and in order. Form is compromised.

Proper exercise form and posture are crucial in neuro gravity resistance training.

Mansfield:

Why train this way?

Fly:

The main purpose of Neuro Gravity Resistance Training is to create new neuro connections between the core muscles and the brain. This training will increase body awareness with newly created neuro connections. The key to create these connections is the amount of time the core is engaged with the build-up of lactic acid as the exercise continues. A long establishment of connection to the core is the main focus of all Neuro Gravity Resistance Training.

Mansfield:

For example, how would I train the chest?

Fly:

Start with a moderate weight, reps will be around fifteen to twenty, but lifting until failure is key. Increasing one's lactic acid tolerance is always the goal. The reason is to activate the nerves within the muscle to enable the body to make a connection that the brain can remember and call upon in times of need. The more nerves that are activated, the more lactic acid that is generated, the better the nervous system can adapt and build the required muscle to handle the work load.

Dumbbell Bench Press: six to seven full reps with flawless posture.

Work the movement with full contraction up and total control on the downward movement and come up until eighty-five percent. Never lock out the arms. Repeat movement until failure. Concentrating on slow reps one second up four seconds down. Again, *flawless posture is essential to success.*

Mansfield:

Why train the chest like this?

Fly: Most of the chest muscles are activated in the lower part of the dumbbell press. The first six inches from your chest out. This is where you have to concentrate to feel that burning lactic acid produced by used glycogen in the pectorals. If you do not have proper posture, it won't even work a little bit.

I suggest a personal trainer teach you proper posture before attempting these exercises.

Mansfield:

What is lactic acid?

Fly:

Let's start at the beginning. When you lift weights or do resistance training, you lift the weight in a range of motion that will bring muscle pain in the areas that are being used most. This is referred to as the burn. The more you resistance train, the higher your individual tolerance for the burn is, the more neuro connections you make. The more connections you make, the closer you get to mind and body becoming one!

The lactic acid burn is a bi-product from the energy used within the specific muscle being trained.

When you first eat carbohydrates, they are converted to energy by the body and it fuels the muscles with a fluid called glycogen. When you begin to use this muscle filled with glycogen, it starts to burn the glycogen for fuel to complete the required set during resistance training. As the fuel is burned up, a bi-product of this glycogen is called lactic acid. It burns within the muscle being trained and tells the brain it must get rid of this toxic chemical as soon as possible. If the lactic acid tolerance is high enough, failure of the movement will occur. This is what we are trying to attain.

Immediately after stopping the movement you begin to breathe hard, bringing oxygen into the lungs which in turn sends oxygen filled blood to the required muscle worked, removes the lactic acid and takes it into the blood stream for processing.

Meanwhile, the body leaves extra blood in the muscle, which actually damages the muscle slightly and it becomes inflamed. The blood stays within the muscle for a while until the trauma is over. This is known as the pump.

Mansfield:

I hung a picture on my wall the other day and now my shoulders are sore.

Fly:

Yes. The soreness is your nervous system already preparing the body for the next time you have to hang a picture and perform that same movement again. If you were to do that every day, your nervous system would adapt to the workload and build the required muscle to accommodate that activity. That's what resistance training is all about.

At the same time your Ego is telling the mind to stop this immediately, it hurts and we don't like that for the body.

Mansfield:

Yes, muscle soreness is what I always looked for the next day after a workout. That's when I knew I had trained well the day before.

Fly:

Every exercise, every rep, must be focused upon, concentrated on and preformed at one hundred and ten percent of your ability, to make the most neuro connections as possible. The more neuro connections you make, the closer you are to mind, body, and soul as one. The closer you are to nature. Nature is always now, as God is.

Mansfield:

So, what is so different about this neuro resistance training?

Fly:

You take weight training, yoga and tai chi and combine those movements with gravity, angles and concentrated breathing and you get *Neuro Resistance Gravity Training*.

Mansfield:

What tools do we need?

Fly

The tools of the nervous system to function at optimum levels are: 1) Exercise, 2) Nutrition 3) Sleep 4) Hydration 5) Optimum Consciousness.

EXERCISE

Exercise is the hardest thing to do, it can hurt and it is the opposite of what our minds tell us to do. Our nervous system is directly connected to our brains and our mind thinks the less the better. The nervous system tells the mind/Ego not to exercise; sit down and relax. Take it easy. The nervous system is only concerned with survival right now. Your mind on the other hand is concerned with past and future and all your experiences. So, it becomes easy to listen to the mind saying, "Relax, got to rest for tomorrow." Meanwhile, the nervous system, which is the great adapter, complies and you get weaker and you lose muscle mass. Your nervous system adapts to the work load. The longer you go without exercise, the weaker you become.

When humans were just starting out, they exercised all day. They had too. They had to eat. So they hunted and gathered for survival. This is our true nature. Now in today's world, technology has made everything easier. We don't even need to walk anymore. There are carts for people with ailments, escalators that are flat along the ground so you don't have to even lift your feet. There are remotes to control your life while sitting and of course, the smart phone. Our lives are so easy now. Why are we so unhealthy, why are we so miserable and depressed?

With all the toxins in our environment and all the preservatives in our food, all the cortisol (stress) that flows through our bodies needs to escape. It needs to be processed and excreted out of the healthy body. Exercise is the way to get it out of the body in large quantities. Otherwise it has nowhere to go, so the nervous system starts to fail, sickness occurs and over long periods of time, it can develop into cancers.

Mansfield:
How much exercise?
Fly:
We need to exercise forty-five minutes to an hour, six days a week.

Mansfield:

What kind of exercise?

Fly:

The kind of exercise should include heavy core muscle activation with conscious thought of muscle being used and required. A *mind to muscle* or neuro connection is the main goal to strengthen the core brain neuro connection. This is the base of all your health. The mind body connection should be strong. Your receiver of energy from throughout the universe will work efficiently, bringing mind and body closer, on a more conscious level.

Mansfield:

What exercises activate the core the most?

Fly:

Core oriented weight lifting, (Neuro Gravity Resistance Training):

Yoga

Par-Core

Obstacle course training.

Tai Chi

Martial Arts

You have to activate your core muscles which are mostly connected from your spine outwards and up to the brain. The brain is the centre of your receiver of energy. It needs to keep those connections for extended periods of time, with total control and awareness of your levels of strength. You need to pay close attention to the neuro connections to specific muscle groups.

Mansfield:
What is good nutrition?
Fly:
Anything God made before man got a hold of it and tried to make it better.

Mansfield:
Why is nutrition so important?
Fly:
Good nutrition keeps the PH of the blood at optimum levels for the health of the body and the immune system. If the blood is too acidic, fungus and disease can start to grow and the same goes if it is too alkaline. The optimum levels for your blood PH should be in the range of 7.35 to 7.45. Anything below a level of 7.0 is considered to be acidic and acidosis can occur (too much Co_2 in blood

stream). This is when fungus and bacteria grow quickly and mutate into disease. Diet is one of the most important for the immune system. When blood acid levels stay between 7.35 and 7.45, no bacteria or fungus can grow at those levels. The immune system is then at its most efficient state.

Mansfield: How do we keep our levels of PH in that range?

Fly:

Eliminate stress as much as possible. Cortisol can turn the blood acidic.

You need to make sure you are getting enough of the green stuff. The dark green vegetables God made for the human body.

Kale, spinach, broccoli, cucumber, and avocado are the top five foods we must eat every day. Along with exercise, good circadian sleep, hydration, and low stress.

Mansfield:

What is negative for the blood PH?

Fly:

Sugar, caffeine, red meat, stress and alcohol are the five main things that bring your blood into an acidic base, where disease and sickness start to grow. If the blood is acidic for long periods of time, then bacteria can survive and mutate into fungus, which can grow between cells activating more genetic mutations into long term disease. Keep the PH levels alkaline not acidic. No sleep, dehydration, and no exercise also contribute to acidic blood.

Mansfield:

What is the best way to change your diet?

Fly:

You must change your previous conditioning on eating slowly over time. Do not jump into a diet so fast that it is a shock to the system and the psyche. The nervous system will rebel, so will Ego. Stress will be created within the body and it will be counterproductive to what you are trying to do. Train your nervous system to respond without stress. Discipline yourself to eat clean for five days in a row every week (for example, Monday – Friday), then reward yourself with whatever you desire for food for two days a week (Saturday and Sunday). Do this and over time you will notice a large change in energy levels, sleep, stress and overall more control over Ego.

With you taking control of your diet, you become aware of Ego even more and start to learn how to control it through basic dieting.

That being said, does it not make sense that nutrition can become a cure for ailments? It has been proven already, as we all know. More and more people have been moving away from pharmaceutical solutions and moving toward a more natural cure from the earth, which would include preventative medicine through natural foods. If you feed the machine the proper fuel it was required to burn from day one, you maximize its potential. In order to maximize potential through nutrition you will also require maximum healing time in sleep.

Sleep

Mansfield:
How much sleep do I need?
Fly:
It is an ongoing learning process to determine how much sleep you need. A good way to track sleep is to not use an alarm and create a plan to go to bed at the same time everyday and awake without an alarm, to find your

bodies' natural clock, while still monitoring daily activity levels.

The more core muscle built, the more neuro connections made, the closer you come to nature. The closer you get to nature and the universe, the more your sleep patterns begin to coincide with the way animals sleep. Bed when it gets dark, up at sunrise.

Sleep is the foundation of healing for the body. The nervous system triggers healing while sleep occurs. Hormones and healing of soft tissue are hard at work while the body sleeps.

Theta is the first stage of sleep (first ten to fifteen minutes of falling asleep), just before you enter REM sleep, your dreaming state. From there you go into a deep sleep (delta brain wave's) enabling the body's healing power according to the tools it has as far as correct nutrition, exercise, hydration, and stress levels. If all these levels are at a good enough level to keep the blood at a correct PH level, then healing will be optimum.

If one particular activity is lacking for the lifestyle, then reaching the correct healing sleep gets more and more difficult. Each individual has a different clock for the amount of sleep that is required for that specific individual. This is labelled as your circadian sleep cycle.

A routine for sleep should be followed every day, same time to bed same time to get up, same amount of sleep per night, if possible. This helps the nervous system regulate hormones throughout the day along with adrenal output and digestion. Therefore, when sleeping, healing is more efficient and quicker.

If nutrients are limited or there has been no exercise, de-hydration, high stresses, the body has to work that much harder and healing will take longer. The immune system could get compromised and sickness could occur.

Hydration:

Mansfield:
How much fluids are needed?
Fly:
The human body is ninety percent water. Without it you die. Drink water to make all other functions of the body work properly. Our bodies are primarily liquid that is taken in and excreted; a constant import and export of fluid. Therefore, it makes sense to maximize the H2O levels needed for all functions to efficiently perform their jobs.

When dehydrated, water is transported from the muscle tissue and sent to the organs for survival. This is our friend the nervous system making sure of survival. But this leaves the body weak and the mind slow. Lack of fluid in the body compromises all aspects of health. Without hydration death occurs within two to three days.

Mansfield:

I didn't know it was all so connected. The food, drink, sleep, exercise and how you think, it's starting to make scents.

Fly:

Now is the time to take you on your journey, a snapshot of a few pieces of your puzzle. As you remember them, all that we have discussed so far will make more sense to you. Tell me about how you grew up?

Stephen Gregory Brown

Book 2

Stephen Gregory Brown

Accounts of a Fly on the wall

(It Was What It Was)

Stephen Gregory Brown

Parents, Asthma, and "Make That Second Effort"

Mansfield:

When I was growing up, I was blessed with a mother and father who loved me, cared for me, and conditioned me to be kind and accountable for my actions.

My father, Bob, came from a small northern Ontario town called Iroquois Falls, Ontario. He left home at seventeen years of age to move to Hamilton, Ontario, to play Major Jr. A hockey for the Hamilton Tiger Cubs. It was 1957 and was the first time he had been away from home. The Detroit Red Wings invited him to Hamilton to try out and he made the team.

When I was a kid, old enough to know what hockey was, my father would tell me old stories about some of the players he once played with and against: Stan Makita, Pat Quinn and Andy Brown to name a few.

He told me of a story of when he was playing against Stan Makita, an NHL Hall Of Famer, who once tried to cream him into the boards in a game in the old Hamilton Forum on Barton St E. on February 12th, 1959.

It was well documented that Makita was more known for his fists than his game, back then.

My dad said, "The St. Catharines team dumped the puck deep in my corner and I was in hot pursuit. Makita thought I didn't see him and he tried to line me up and put me out of the game. Little did he know, I did see him coming, made some adjustments and ducked just at the last moment."

Makita went for the hit and missed. He ended up separating his shoulder on the play and was out for a number of weeks. When this Hall of Famer hockey player mentions this in his book, *I Play to Win* he mentions the injury to his shoulder like this. He says, "someone threw a dime on the ice" and he states that is what he slipped on and how he hurt his shoulder. My Dad knew the truth. He says there was no dime on the ice. My dad just outsmarted him in that particular moment in time.

Fly:

That Hall of Famer was saving his true insecurities and protecting self through his Ego, by saying there was a dime on the ice and that is what made him fall into the boards and injure his shoulder.

Mansfield:

When I was growing up, my father always struck me as a kind man who wa everyone's friend. He knew a lot a people around town, at least I thought he knew a lot of people, but I was only young.

He was an athlete. It was a normal thing for him to play road hockey with me as well as baseball, football, soccer and even go running. Everything was physical activities. He played these games with me, just because he loved to do these activities himself. It was clear to me even at a young age, that I had his genetics and gift of athleticism.

As I grew and became more athletic I was conditioned by my father and society to compete all the time. Every athletic event I tried my best and seemed to excel in anything that I tried. I just had to mimic or copy what I saw and it would all work out. Before I knew it, I was excelling at whatever I put my mind to.

My father would feed my self esteem, build my Ego for the future and train me to survive out in the world. Basically, he was my mentor. He was my hero, and still is. Without my father, I would be the kind of person I am today.

When I was in my third year of ice hockey at age eight my father became my hockey coach. He trained me to get thick skin" which means don't let words hurt you.

He would say "I don't want excuses, I want results", which translates to, "just get the job done!" This was ingrained in my mind when I was having an asthma attack on the ice in practise and couldn't skate as fast as when I had full lung capacity. This saying has always stuck with me and brings back memories of emotional pain as a child, but that experience made me more emotionally tough simply because I got through it.

On the other side of it, my father always praised me when a job was well done. He gave me positive encouragement and supported me when I really needed it. All the positive encouragement and praise my father gave me was even more of an influence on my Ego. I believed it when he told me I was good and that I had so much potential. I also believed him when he told me when I didn't do well.

He praised me on the many goals that I scored or assisted on in hockey and being a kid, (and where my Ego's development was at the time), I was always trying to reach for perfection. This meant I had to be perfect for my father which made me remember those words, "I don't want excuses, I want results" all my life.

The funny thing was my father would always say, and still does to this day, "Always do the absolute best that you can and I will be proud of you".

Fly:

This is how a young Ego is developed. It is conditioned to the environment around it. That is why it is so important for children to have good positive role models that teach within truth.

Mansfield:

The way I thought, was that every game that he saw me play, I needed his approval. My Ego and self esteem depended on it.

I know that I hung on every word my father said. I trusted him. I desperately needed his approval on any athletic activity. I would always be concerned about how I played. He was ultimately in charge of developing my Ego and self esteem. Sometimes when I didn't play well, he would tell me and it would break my confidence and I believe that it affected me emotionally, because at a young age I associated my father's love with my ability to perform in sports and win his approval.

Fly:

At least that's what Ego thought, but there was a true feeling that had no words deep inside the psyche. Your father loved you no matter what. At the time, being a young kid, you would always listen to Ego rather than your true feelings and intuitions. Everything you had learned was all through Ego via beta consciousness, so those feelings you had towards your father were that of love, but also of anger if he said you didn't play well. He could control your whole mental state with only a few words.

Mansfield:

There were times after a game that where so emotional to me like when, my father expressed that I didn't play as well as I could have, I thought the world was going to end. I needed to get out on the ice and prove myself to him. When I got mad, I got better and worked harder. He realized this and used it to better me. I hated him at the time. I thought he wouldn't love me if I wasn't good and maintained his approval.

Now looking back, I am so grateful for him doing what he did. At that time in my life, he being a hockey coach, he was learning, reading and living *Vince Lombardi* rules. He would always be quoting Lombardi in our private game plans before a hockey game on the way to the rink. It made me more mentally tough, but emotionally fragile.

My old man built my Ego and he knew what he was doing. He wanted me to never be satisfied. Never give in. Never quit and I believed it all.

In sports, if you do the work, it will always pay off, eventually. But at that time, as an eight to eighteen-year-old boy, when you are learning to be a man, any experiences, any role models, any influences, end up building your Ego into the mask that you determine to be your identity. My mask, early on in life, was that of a hockey player, because my dad was a hockey player and his approval was all I cared about. It didn't only include hockey, it carried over to all the other sports I played throughout high school. Every sport I tried I needed to excel in and gain my father's approval.

Fly:

It seems just yesterday that all this was going on in our head, but now I realize how we were conditioned. We are so vulnerable when we are young. Our minds absorb energy, through our thoughts on what we see, feel, hear, taste and smell. Those are also associated with emotions, which have a physical reaction within the body, releasing chemicals and hormones, endorphins and dopamine, all connected to each experience and storing it in Ego for future use. This is how a personality is developed. This is how an Ego is programmed.

Building Integrity

Mansfield:

I remembered how my father contributed building my integrity when I was nine years old.

My friend and I were in grade four. We wanted to be like the older kids on the block who smoked cigarettes. We thought they were so cool. They were in grade six and all the girls liked these guys. So, my friend Paul and I would pick up old butts on the street and light them with lighters we had shoplifted at the grocery store.

One day I had put one of the lighters in my top drawer in my room. I still remember it as if it was yesterday. It was a Saturday morning and my sister and I usually got up to watch cartoons with a bowl of cereal. It was every kid's ritual on a Saturday morning.

As I came down the stairs into the kitchen and got my bowl, I noticed on the dresser was a lighter. Same color as the one I had in my drawer.

I ran back upstairs to my room to check.

Yep, it was mine! Why was it there? Oh no. What do I do?

My parents were still sleeping and all that I had to do was sit and wait until they got up, to see where this would lead.

When mom and dad got up, it was as any Saturday morning. We were happy it was the weekend and ready for breakfast.

I was watching TV downstairs when I got the call from my dad. "Come up here please."

I came up and was asked the question. "Your mother found this in your drawer. Where did you get it?

I replied, "Found it."

Dad says, "Where?"

I said, "The dead end."

He said "Who was you with?

I said, "Paul."

My dad then asked, "What are you guys doing with a lighter at your age?

I shot back, "Just for camp fires in the woods," not even looking up from my second bowl of cereal.

"Ok, no problem, give me Paul's number and I'll ask him myself. If your story doesn't match, and your lying to me, you are in way more trouble than if you tell me the truth now."

I caved in and told him we stole it from the grocery store.

"Who else did you steal from?" said my dad.

"The variety store up the street." I replied.

That day my father gave me a choice for punishment. I could either take two weeks grounding in the middle of summer vacation or go to the variety store return the lighter, confess to my crime and pay the owners for all the things I stole over that summer.

He asked me: "How much do you owe them?"

I replied "Ten bucks in chocolate bars."

I chose to return the lighter and pay for the chocolate.

Fly:

Your Ego thought, if that's all the punishment you were going to get, you would be getting off pretty easy.

Mansfield:

He took me to that big grocery store and made me ask for the manager all by myself at nine years old. I had to explain what I did and apologize. Then I had to go to the variety store and do the same thing. I recall it was the hardest thing I had to do up until that day of my life. I had to face an adult, admit I was wrong and ask for forgiveness. It was hard and a lesson for my developing Ego. It humbled me.

I did it, and fought my dad all the way. I whined and cried all the way there. It was scary being in unfamiliar territory in life at that time.

When it was all said and done, I still got grounded for two weeks of summer vacation, the most boring two weeks of my young life. My grounding was so strict: I could not leave the property or watch TV. I had to be in the moment for two weeks. That's how I was punished. It left an impression on my Ego to never steal again. It made me always think, "if I do this, what is the worst that could happen?" That lesson stuck with me all my life. It made me think of having to be accountable for my actions.

Fly:

It is amazing how with experience in developing your Ego, your punishment really was to be in the moment all the time. That's what Ego hates, so it was either find something else to occupy Ego or have Ego be so bored, you will never do it again.

Mansfield:

I remember occupying my time during that grounding by riding my bike around our lot for hours because I couldn't leave the property. So I rode my bike around and around the 108' x 60' lot of grass. Two weeks of that and I got in more trouble for wearing a bike path in the grass around the house.

Fly:

That was extremely boring for Ego. I remember you getting so mad and frustrated that summer. That punishment stuck with you the rest of your life.

If your father had just made you return the items and pay for them without the two-week grounding, it wouldn't have taught you accountability and we know you probably would have continued to steal.

The Only Marilyn I Ever Knew

Mansfield:

My mother Marilyn cared for me through all my asthma attacks as a kid. She cared for me when I had pneumonia, seven times before grade six. The biggest contribution my mother ever made to my personality was her compassion and love for me. How she loved me, helped me to realize what love really was. It took self fifty years to define love and get over all the conditioning that is the world. My mother's love was unconditional, as Jesus' love was, as my love for my children is.

My mother would always take the time to explain where I went wrong and teach me about consequences. She would always make me follow through with my punishments for doing wrong. She never got soft and let me off. She taught me to think before I act. She was the best nurturer. I am so grateful for all her lessons.

I remember she was, and still is, the kind of mother that reads something in the paper cuts it out and wants you to read it. This small lesson, in a newspaper article, was for our future reference and to educate us on the world that was outside. She still cuts out newspaper articles for me and keeps them for our weekly visits. I used to hate the articles and was too impatient to read. Now I still have no patience, but I always do what my mother says and deep down I really love it. She taught me so much.

My mother and I seem to be on the same frequency in the universe. She is so easy to talk to and understood who I was before I knew who I was, at times.

I get my creative side from her. I was always involved in sports as a kid. Athletics were my play time. I was very creative when playing sports. That is when I would get lost in alpha consciousness and excel at sports.

The other creative side I developed later on in life. These were things that had to do with the arts.

Mom always told me I had a knack for poetry because my grade four teacher phoned home and told my mother to encourage me to continue pursuing this field as I had a talent for it.

I remember my mother telling me this and feeling that if I did poetry, all the guys would laugh and make fun of me. There was a guy in my class that was a dancer. All the guys that played sports made fun of this guy. I didn't want to be like him! So I put it out of my mind. I was building an image, a mask, a role as an elite athlete. A hockey star/basketball star type mask, that was kind, considerate of others, open minded and forgiving. That's what I was going for anyway.

Now being fifty years old I am still that grade four kid playing those roles to some extent, but with so many more layers of experience. The dramas in my life are now just moments in time that need to be dealt with. I thank my mother for this.

As my personality grew, my Ego grew with every success. I had a certain mask that I used throughout high school. The role of an athlete was my choice. You know, the nerds, the athletes, the stoner's, the artiste's, Goth's, etc. Everyone had a mask. Everyone just wanted to fit in somewhere.

Fly:

High school developed your Ego as it did everyone's. You were tall, good looking and an athlete, not interested in the school work, just the sports, babes and parties. You had a fifty-five percent average throughout, and were so insecure, you were always looking for compliments, or Ego boosts all the time. You always had a girlfriend, because self needed one.

True self would say, "Yeah we need a woman to love".

Ego, trying to fulfill Maslow's physiological needs would say "I need sex," so Ego and self compromised.

This is why you always had to have a girlfriend. It feed you the love energy your body craved and it satisfied Ego with the sex. That is why sex, Ego and true self can get confusing in adolescents. Sex and Ego go hand in hand until one can get over his or her conditioning and truly love unconditionally.

Sports and Consciousness

Mansfield:

Basketball and hockey where my main sports in high school and soccer in the summer. Those were my activities all the time. As a child and young adult, I would play sports as entertainment. These sports always had training regiments and a lot of them would always suggest weight training. This is where it all started. Once I got started on the weights, I enjoyed it. I enjoyed the pump you would get after a hard set. I lifted my first weights when I was nine years-old, would train for hockey between seasons with weights and by fifteen years old weights became a part of everyday life and are still to this day.

As I grew more interested in weight training and my hockey career was coming to an end, the sport of bodybuilding became my main interest at age twenty-one. I had been training regularly for six years and when junior hockey was over at age twenty-one, for some reason I knew I had to continue the competitive Egoic nature that I had been conditioned for. That is all I ever knew to that point in my life.

Fly:

Sports are a wonderful way to train a child to find themselves. Sports are good for their health physically and mentally. When you play sports, it develops a child's Ego in many different ways.

Competition is Ego vs. Ego. Whether it is one on one, or a team sport, it is always the same. This is what different societies all over the world believe.

Sports train a child to work at something to get better. It trains them to give of themselves to benefit the team for a greater good. Sports help a developing mind learn discipline. They help build self esteem within the young, developing Ego.

Mansfield:

I remember I had a huge disagreement over a girl with my teammate in Jr. hockey. We had an argument that almost came to fists. We had a hockey game that night and the argument wasn't finished. We both went on the ice angry.

I was defence, he was the goalie. I knew we would have to work together to make sure the other team didn't score. Even though I was ready to punch his lights out when we were on dry land, now that we were on the ice in a hockey situation, I knew that all that outside, girl crap had nothing to do with now, on the ice. I can remember slapping his goalie pads with my stick and telling him "Let's go man".

He knew what I meant and he said the same back to me. We played that game as if we were best friends still. It didn't matter what happened before. The situation was now and the only way we could win was if we worked together. We had to put our Egos aside and respect and trust each other to accomplish what we needed to do. The team came first. We won the game.

Fly:

Experiences like this one taught us to put selfishness aside and work towards the greater goal of winning that particular game on that particular day. In other words, hockey and sports in general teach you how to discipline your Ego. How to stay in the moment.

Mansfield:

I also noticed while playing sports, that when you are in the heat of the action and are totally consumed within your mind on the task at hand and things are going exactly like you plan it seems like your body is moving fluidly and effortlessly as you succeed at every obstacle. In the 90's they used to call it being in the zone.

Fly:

When you have mind and body as one while performing a physical sport, you change your consciousness to the point of being able to jump from alpha consciousness to beta consciousness at will.

The best players in each sport are the best at finding alpha. They have mastered jumping back and forth to the point of feeling most comfortable in their lives when they are performing their sport.

They achieve this by practise. They practise until all the movements needed to be successful at their particular sport become automatic to the brain. The brain sends signals to each muscle needed to complete a physical movement so many times that it is done without Ego having to be involved.

In other words, they don't have to think, it just happens.

Mansfield:

I have been there while playing sports, but unfortunately not enough. The reason for that is I didn't practise enough to have it become automatic all the time. I didn't know any of this when I was growing up, but being older and wiser, I see where consciousness of now plays such a big role in the moment.

Fly:

When consciousness extends itself when playing a team sport, it can change the energy within a moment. We have all witnessed it within sport, when one team is being dominated by another team and the consciousness of a dominating team changes. They go from not being able to make a mistake to everything going wrong, within a short period of time. The consciousness of the team changes and the energy switches to the team that was being beaten so badly. This is where the comeback starts. The team being beaten so badly gains the momentum and succeeds at winning.

The two different mindsets of winning and losing become habit forming. This is Ego and team conditioning.

Mansfield:

I have lived that change in energy many times while playing sports from both sides. I know what both feel like.

Fly:

When the majority of the team members have had the right nutrition, sleep, hydration, preparation, and discipline, reaching alpha consciousness while playing a sport and winning can be achieved more easily. This is the goal of a championship team and each athlete. Being able to slip in and out of alpha and beta consciousness, almost as if team members can communicate telepathically and anticipate each play. It is when everything slows down physically and each goal is set and achieved within that moment as planned. The manipulation of that energy at that time becomes second nature.

Mansfield:

What do you mean manipulate energy?

Fly:

Everything is energy. Fitness activity is an excellent example of manipulating energy through the body to make it adapt to the work load to make that activity easier for the body to handle.

Humans have been manipulating energy to accomplish things in this world since the beginning of time. Humans build machines to do the work that man used to have to do by hand. In the pursuit of an easier life, humans have neglected manipulating energy through their own exercise. They have become lazy, fat and unhealthy. Their receivers are broken and they can't receive the positive energy needed to heal and live content.

Arnold, Lou and the Flipper

Mansfield:

When I was seven years old, I remember watching wide world of sports, and seeing Lou Ferrigno win the Mr. Universe, Bodybuilding Championship. I immediately asked my father, "How do you get big arms like that guy?" He took me downstairs to our basement and showed me the barbell bicep curl. He told me to do three sets of ten at a weight that was hard to do at that age. I did just that. Two days later I remember complaining to my dad that my arms were sore. He told me that I was building muscle from my workouts and he said, "I should eat my meat. Meat builds muscle."

I started weight training for hockey on a regular basis, when I was fifteen years old, m friend Tim, the goaltender on the team, would weight train two or three times a week in his garage. We would do bench press and curls, then go look at ourselves in the car window which was slightly convex. That window made us look like Lou Ferrigno, the Incredible Hulk. But I was only a skinny kid, six feet, weighing 160lbs. But I liked the way the weights made my arms feel, all swollen and pumped up. I noticed the more I trained my arms the bigger they got. People would comment that I was getting bigger and I liked it. My Ego liked it. It gave me more confidence. I didn't want to lose that so I kept working out. Logically I thought, why stop and lose all the gains. Just stay in two states, of maintenance and growth."

My body was growing and so was my Ego. With Ego, with insecurity, with all that comes with a twenty-two-year-old's psyche, I decided to enter my first bodybuilding show. It was 1988 at a high school in Toronto.

I began training hard for it in August even though the show would be at the end of October. I was a huge fan of

Arnold Swartzenegger, ever since the Conan movies and always had him as my "who I wanted to be like" hero.

I belonged to a gym by now, was living on my own, a bachelor apartment in downtown Hamilton. I had met many people through the gyms and made some acquaintances who sold steroids and this is when my Ego decided to step over the line. I purchased a small amount of oral steroids and some testosterone to inject into your my shoulder to get ready for the show.

As the show approached, I was working construction in Toronto, lining water mains. I was tall and strong so they had me setting up temporary water mains while the existing ones were repaired. It was physical and then I had to hit the gym afterwards. They were long days. Six-thirty in the morning on the road, home by six at night, then to the gym. I had conditioned myself to do it, day in and day out. This is where I learned to train my Ego. I resisted bad foods that everyone else would eat. I would go to the gym on a Friday night to train instead of going out to bars and chase women. That could all wait till after I won my show. As Ego thought. Ego was not going to give in. It had a plan and was going to stick to it.

Self thought "Oh my God, I am a drug addict, sticking needles in me. I am a junky. This is not me. I was not raised like this. This goes against everything that was taught to me."

Fly:

Yes, self felt that and needed to go through all of that Ego stuff and come out the other end still in one piece mentally and physically.

This was your conflict throughout life. Ego always wins until you realize that Ego can't hurt you if you are aware of it. If you decide you are not your conditioning. Your conditioning is your Ego. Self takes over the vessel once self realizes Ego will never be satisfied. When this occurs, true self looks for another way.

As I told you, as does the Bible, your Ego is your devil. Submit to the universe, which is now. It is what it is, it was what it was and it will be what it will be. We are all now, we are all everything, we are all one.

Mansfield:

I now say that every day to remind myself that nothing really matters because all we really have is right now. That is all we have ever had. Be in the moment give one hundred percent and tomorrow will take care of itself.

As my bodybuilding increased, my identity shifted to bodybuilder from athlete. I had been taking steroids pretty steady after that first show (which I placed fourth in). I had got my weight up to 245lbs by October of 1989. This is when I met my first wife. I can remember the feelings I had with her. Her voice was like a sweet song bird that relaxed my soul. I knew I liked to be with only one woman at a time, my Ego would give in to self there. It just made it easier to build muscle, if you didn't have to deal with the loneliness issues and the love issues. As I said, love is always a choice. My main goal at the time was to be a pro bodybuilder. So much so that I heard through the boys at the gym that you should inject steroids into your glutes, (rear end) because it is the biggest muscle group on the body and it will have a better effect.

So I started to inject my glutes with anabolic steroids. Not having any training or guidance I decided to do the first shot at work where I was a material handler working afternoons. I was able to pick this shift because I would be the only one of our department working, so I had the time to run to the washroom and take my shot.

When I did, I injected too low in the gluteus maximus (rear end) and caught the sciatic nerve. I was in great pain. I had to leave work. I had to drive twenty-three kilometers home and go to a hospital. It was the most excruciating pain ever felt up to this point in my life. I was puking up my dinner, sweating and the muscles around the damaged nerve were into spasm.

I remember the debate in my head that day before I took the shot.

Fly:

Wait until you can get someone to show you how to inject your glute, so you don't hurt anything.

Mansfield:

No, I need to get big now. That could take a week; can't stop the cycle; must train hard and win. Do it now, it'll be alright.

Fly:

I remember, you were all Ego, no patience. You were twenty-three years old.

Mansfield:

I spent that night in the hospital loaded with pain killers. The outside of my foot had gone numb and I could not control the downward action of my foot when I walked. All my pain was in my foot and shin. The doctor at the time said it was nerve damage and I might not ever gain that mobility back again. It would all need time to heal. I remember the doctor saying that the nerve regeneration would take one year for every one eighth of an inch damaged. I injected in the middle of my ass and my foot was where the pain was. That is almost a meter of nerve to heal.

Fly:

When they told you that you might never gain the feeling back in your foot, you didn't believe them for one second. You knew how you felt and your mind, run by your Ego, would not believe you would be this way the rest of your life.

Mansfield:

I walked as if I had a floppy foot. The gym guys would call me flipper because it would flip and flop when I walked and slap the ground. They were just having fun with me. The funny thing was that as my workouts went on, within half an hour, the pain would be gone from my foot and I had more control over the flapping and slapping of my foot on the ground as I walked. This is when I started to realize that exercise can heal the body through hormone release and endorphins. The more intense the exercise, the less pain I felt in my foot. This ultimately took fifteen years to heal to the point where I would have full control and no pain in that area again. I was lucky and I attribute all the intense exercise for the recovery by always having positive hormones and endorphins running through the system daily.

Fly:

When you love someone and the love is returned, your receiver (the body) produces hormones that are more beneficial to the body. These positive hormones to the body increases immune, health and healing.

If there is no way for the body to express love and this state keeps up for a long period of time, physical heath will eventually be compromised. The electromagnetic frequency of the receiver, (body) when giving and receiving love on a regular basis, is where our human bodies need to be to achieve optimum health, mind and body. The human psyche depends on love for survival of the species.

Mansfield:

My first wife went through all that nerve damage from steroids with me and she stuck by me. I give her credit for that especially. We weren't even married and she stuck by me.

We met in October of '89 and were married the following year, October 1990. At that time I was working at an air craft landing gear manufacturer, working as a material handler, moving aircraft parts from one process to next. It was a job that had me moving around on my feet for eight hours a day. But my Ego had to build muscle so I quit that November. I was unemployed and was two months into a marriage. My Ego thought I was better than this.

I was unemployed, married, living in a bachelor apartment with my wife and two cats. I was a bodybuilder, and that's what my Ego wanted me to portray. That's who I was. I made money bouncing in night clubs, working security for concerts and sporting events and took jobs for short periods of time to see if there was something else I could do and find an interest. My Ego just didn't like working.

My next show was in 1991. I was definitely in better shape for that show than the previous one. I was still taking steroids, still Ego as big as ever. I came in fourth again out of a field of eleven. A good showing in my gym community. I was accepted as a "Competitive Bodybuilder" in my gym, one that the former Mr. Canada owned.

Mindfulness of a Fly on the Wall

Layers of Life

Fly:

That brings the story to the next chapter or layer. See, everything in life seems to overlap. There are no straight cuts. Layers and layers of things overlapping and connecting to each other. Life is a symphony of layers of experiences. Pay attention and the song will sound clearer and more precise sooner than later. Get caught up in your own Ego and the daily drama that happens and you will miss the hidden meanings of what you are supposed to learn from that experience.

Mansfield:

Now my unemployment insurance is about to run out. I need a job. So I decide to take a job selling memberships at my gym in August, 1991. I had never had a sales job before, so I thought "What the heck?" I am in the gym all day anyway so why not get paid to be there, right?

Fly:

Right. You learned how to sell from the guy that trained you. He was a master of the visual sale. The grand tour. The open-ended questions that would make a person communicate with their body and tones. That would enable him to find the hot buttons on why they wanted to join this gym. This was your first sales job. You did well. When they realized how much money you were making, they cut back on how much commission could be made. You didn't like that.

Mansfield:

I had worked at the gym for eight months and decided I (Ego) was bored selling memberships and wanted to sell at a higher commission sales job. I had mastered selling memberships, but the hours were long if you wanted to make good money. I wanted a job with the least amount of effort for the biggest pay off.

I learned from my job at the gym to copy the tones and body language of my trainers. I watched them in action. Watched what made them successful and just copied them. I paid special attention to the detail of their questions to the customers and how they would always bring it back to "If I could do this for you, would you buy it right now?" I learned how to say that in so many different ways that you could close a sale, or know the buying signals, so that you could make a living at it. I liked sales because it was like scoring a goal in hockey. There was nothing like scoring a goal in hockey. That's what sales had become to me.

Fly:

Deep down, you knew sales weren't what your purpose was, or what you were supposed to do, but it was working for the moment.

Mansfield:

I was now making pretty good money and had decided to get a personal trainer. The cost was an initial $300 down and $75 per month. The trainer lived in London and Toronto. I lived in Hamilton. There was no internet at the time, so we would travel every second weekend to be assessed by the trainer on our look and how to train. It was a fun time in my life because of all the hope of success. Everyone that trained with this trainer would win shows. He was an awesome trainer and his girlfriend was already a professional women's bodybuilder. The exercise knowledge he possessed was like no other of his time. What I learned from them was the base of *Neuro Gravity Resistance Training.*

My wife wasn't all that keen on the trainer because of the money we had to give this guy and his girlfriend. But both of the trainers were well known.

So she said "Everything you spend on training and steroids, I get to spend on shopping." I agreed. I was going pro!

I gained knowledge from the trainers from London and Toronto. I had gotten my weight up to 310lbs; a mass of walking muscle and fat. I looked like a huge wrestler, not a bodybuilder. That was their plan, to get as big as possible and then lose all the fat, keeping as much muscle as possible.

Six months went by, and the $75 a month was becoming too much for our budget. I had to drop the trainer. I was on my own.

I was on my own for the show that was only three months away. But I had learned from the trainers and the other guys training with them and had gone through the contest prep stage of training. This was what I had to go on.

I went from 310lbs to 225lbs in six months of contest dieting.

Fly:

Yes! you couldn't wait to lose all that extra fat you carried. You liked the discipline of the diet with a date set for a show. Ego was so obsessed with keeping muscle and looking big, you stressed ten pounds of muscle off in the last three months without the trainers. You worried and stressed way too much. It created loads of cortisol that would eat away at the muscle you had worked so hard to build. You weighed in at 225lbs the day of the show and came third out of nine competitors.

If I can get it for you in blue, would you buy the car?

Mansfield:

That's when I changed sales jobs to make more money to buy more steroids and become a pro bodybuilder. I became a car salesman to continue my lifestyle, really not knowing what things I would learn from all this. Looking back, my Ego was totally in the driver seat of the vessel. I remember mimicking my manager, watching him make car deals, watching his actions, body language, and tone. Seeing his smile at just the right time to make people warm up to you. Make them trust you quickly.

I copied it all and made it my own. My mask now was the salesmen/bodybuilder. The bodybuilding made great conversation in the showroom. Car sales seemed challenging, but I always remained humble so I could learn from the best guys. They were always respected no matter how much of a dick they could be at times. I knew you had to work their Egos a bit to get them to help you. They sold cars and that's all that counted in that business.

I was re-conditioning my thinking by doing something that I remember saying to myself when I was 18 years old. "I would never be a commission salesman because you never know when you will get paid"

Now I was living on commissions. I was successful at it. I retrained myself to do something I was terrified of doing. I was able to make a living for three years at selling cars.

Fly:

Then Ego got bored again. Ego is always getting bored. It always needs to be entertained with drama.

Ego always needs more money, better this, and a lot more of that!

Mansfield:

The Year was 1995; I changed sales jobs again and decided to sell photo copiers, fax machines and other office equipment. I used the same formula to learn the business. It had seemed to work before, so why not again?

I mimicked my trainer, who was also my boss. I learned the business quick enough to win sales trips, contests and qualify for bonuses. The money was good. My Ego grew. My confidence grew.

The new job included training. I had to go for mandatory training at a hotel in Toronto for two business days. We had to show our product knowledge and demonstration skills on the equipment.

Most of the first day was all product knowledge and how to do a presentation, paperwork etc. The second day we were to be scored on a demonstration presentation and the results would be published to the home branch.

The first day went great. I met some other sales trainees and we went out for dinner. We were walking back to the hotel so we all had a few drinks that night and were pretty late getting back to the room. I remember sitting in a diner eating a hamburger and spilling mustard down my shirt and not caring.

The next morning, which I think was only three hours later, came quick. I got up and still felt intoxicated. I had a headache, but nothing too bad. I took some Tylenol and got ready for work. We had to be in the conference room of the hotel at eight in the morning. It was just on the first floor of the hotel. It was seven-thirty and I was awake and dressed. I start chugging coffee and tried to eat a donut, but my stomach was having nothing to do with food.

The class of thirty reps from around the Province of Ontario started their presentations on the photocopier. One by one they proceeded up on to the stage and presented their demo. Meanwhile I was not feeling so good. Hung over like no tomorrow, my head pounding and I felt nauseous.

Just then, the instructor called me up to do my presentation.

Oh no! Why me? Now? I am in panic mode! My Ego is trying to save me.

I then pleaded with the instructor to let me use the washroom first, as I wasn't feeling well. I exited quickly out the door and proceeded to the washroom. It was at the other end of the longest hall in the world! It had to be a football field away, or so it seemed. All I could see was this little Hertz® rental car guy sitting at his booth all alone at the end of the hall were the washrooms where. It was eight-fifteen or so.

I felt it in my stomach. I started to jog, then run, then an all-out sprint! I was a 310lb bodybuilder in a suit and tie, sprinting to go throw up in the washroom in a fancy hotel lobby on a business trip and I was to be graded on my performance on a presentation of a photocopier.

BARF! BARF! Barf! I was sprinting down the corridor of this nice hotel, puking and running into it. As I look up I see the rental car guy watching in amazement. I have never seen a look on someone's face like he had on his. He was watching a fat, 310lb bodybuilder running full speed into his own puke.

By the time I got to the washroom and bent over the toilet, all the puke was gone. I had no puke to give that toilet. At that exact moment, I thought to myself, "I am so fired for this. I suck. I am a looser! What do I tell my boss? My wife? Where will I work now?" A million questions and answers went through my head.

Fly:

You now know that that was just Ego panicking with all this drama. But then I stepped in and made you go look at the damage in the mirror. What did you look like?

Mansfield:

Huh? I don't look too bad? All the puke was just water and some coffee, couldn't eat this morning so it is all just liquid in and liquid out. All the puke was on my shirt and tie. If I did my suit jacket up, I could hide the puke stains. So that is just what I did. Since I had puked I was feeling better. Maybe I could pull this off, I thought.

I dried my face off, gained composure and walked back into the training room. The instructor asked if I was ok and ready to proceed. I took a deep breath and said "Yes."

As I walk up to the stage, all 310lb of me sweating in my suit, feeling faint, I feel like I am going to puke again! What do I do?

I walked up on stage and saw there was a door at the side in the middle on the right end of the stage. The photocopier is in the middle of the stage. I was definitely going to puke again, so I walked through the door on the right side of the stage and found it was a closet. I was in there a good 10 seconds that seemed like an hour.

As I stood in the closet on the stage, all alone, getting ready for the embarrassment of walking out with the entire training class watching.

Fly:

I remember you having two choices. Give up and quit, say you are sick and maybe you would be excused, or suck it up and go do the presentation. Your conditioning from your father's teaching you "quitters never win and winners never quit" sets in. That is integrity conditioning of your Ego and that is what you did.

Mansfield:

I ran out of the closet and immediately started my presentation. I presented the SF 2022-photocopier to the best of my hungover ability and got a seventy-five percent grade. Suit done up of course.

I thought I had gotten away with it until, as we were all walking down the hall leaving for lunch, the instructor says out loud, "I think someone was sick out here, it smells real bad". A trainee says "Yeah, I think it was Mansfield".

That was all I heard of it until I got back to work the next week. The instructor reported me to my boss, but recommended that these things happen once in a while in the industry. I passed and didn't quit and was warned not to do it again. I was also selling a lot of photocopiers so my boss could easily forget it and move on. I was lucky. Nothing like that ever happened again. Live and Learn.

Stephen Gregory Brown

Love, Ego, and "I am not one of those guys'

Fly::

With layers of experience each decision creates new paths and choices.

Mansfield:

The year is 1995. I am looking for justification as to who I am, and who I think I am. The character I have created in my version of who I am is not getting the justification I need from my wife of five years.

At that time I needed to be acknowledged and keep living my fantasy life I think I am living, that of a bodybuilder. I was still doing steroids, looking good in my eyes and needing acknowledgement. Not from my wife but others, especially females.

Fly:

Ego always needs to be acknowledged, justified, convinced and in control, until you realize that it all just doesn't matter. No one gives a shit who you think you are because they are trying to figure out who they are.

Mansfield:

This is when I began to cheat on my wife.

There was a girl from the gym I would fool around with on occasion, a girl from the dealership I would too. It was the third time I cheated that I got caught.

Fly:

All these decisions were from the Ego part of your mind that was trying to justify your actions. Ego constantly needed someone who could appreciate all your hard work in the gym and at work. Ego needed always needed a boost because you were so insecure. The cheating was exciting, but the guilt (self) would in turn drive you crazy.

That wasn't you either. Just like the steroids you continued to do. You did these things, knowing clearly that it was destructive to, not only to your own psyche, but also to your marriage.

Mansfield:

After the first night of cheating on my wife with a girl whose last name I didn't even know, I knew deep down once I crossed that line, the marriage was over. My conditioning was that once you marry, you marry for life, like my parents. This was me getting over a small portion of my conditioning.

We separated by the end of the year, as she caught me at one of the ladies houses I was seeing on the side. We had had a fight the night before and I told her I was staying at a friend's. A mutual friend spotted my car in the parking lot of the girl I was messing around with and informed my wife. I found a note on my car the next morning when I left the girl's apartment. "It's over!" it said. That was the end.

Fly:

Your big Ego ruined that marriage and your insecurity created that marriage.

Your parents, who were married at age twenty-one, put pressure on you to find a nice girl and settle down. In almost a way of having your father's approval of the bodybuilding and your lifestyle, you remember vividly deciding to marry for two reasons: Your parent's approval and the decision to love someone to cure the loneliness you felt at that age. You wanted to be different and needed to love someone. That is when you felt right. When you were loving someone and they were in accordance with your Ego, but weren't conscious of these thoughts at the time. It was more a feeling than a thought put into words. That feeling was me the Fly.

Mansfield:

So what did I do? I was a dumbass. I moved in with the girl I got caught with. She offered me free rent until I got on my feet again. Big mistake! All Ego. That didn't last very long and when it was over she demanded three grand in back rent and would stalk me for a whole two years. I paid off my debt and there was no excuse for her to see or talk to me again. That was a layer of experience that I learned from. I never cheated on a women ever again. I didn't like the guilt and negative energy it made my Ego produce. The cheating created worry and anxiety about hurting my wife and covering my tracks with lies. There was absolutely nothing positive about cheating on a mate because the Ego boosts were only temporary. They were all an illusion of my mind.

Fly:

Cheating is an insecure Ego desperately looking to be justified. The more insecure an Ego is, the more it looks for validation on its' own development. The Ego will justify any action by round about logic that convinces self it is the right thing to do.

Mansfield:

June 1996: I meet my next wife at a bar we both frequented at the time. Still a bodybuilder, still competing, still doing steroids, but knowing I wouldn't become a pro bodybuilder. I didn't want to do the quantities of steroids that were required to become pro. I still stayed on the steroids because I liked how they made me look and feel. I never did large cycles because I was blessed to not ever be able to afford it. I was always with someone in a relationship because I needed both bodybuilding and a place to express my love so I wouldn't be lonely. I would not give up either.

My next wife was four years older, blond, beautiful, very nice and friendly to everyone. She could party. That's where I was at this point in my life. Parties every weekend, eat and drink like crazy; just fun.

Fly:

Once you realized the pro bodybuilding dream was over, you switched your mask to bodybuilder/actor. You became a professional actor, mainly because one day in a conversation as you were boasting about your sales successes to your father, he said, "Why don't you become an actor? You're such a good salesman. I bet you could be a good actor."

So you did. Mainly to make your father proud. Again with the fatherly approval.

You heard the money was good and they were filming in Toronto all the time. This is where Ego justified your bodybuilding workouts and continuing with the steroids to get acting parts so you could follow in Arnold's footsteps as a bodybuilder turned actor. You ended up being successful in acting, getting four to five gigs a year to supplement your sales career.

Mansfield:

I was now selling industrial supplies and equipment, which I would continue to do for nine years. It was a steady salary, plus commission. I thought I was the man.

Fly:

That was Ego! Hot wife, good money, partying with beautiful people every weekend. What a lifestyle.

Mansfield:

We lived together for two years and decided to marry. She originally said she didn't want kids, but two years into the marriage she wanted to adopt. We adopted three wonderful kids from a town nearby. They were fraternal: brother and sisters, two girls and a boy.

Fly:

Yes, that is what we talked about earlier. Their conditioning was poorly done to the point of being taken away from their fraternal parents. They were neglected children who never had a stable home.

Mansfield:

We raised the children together for seven years before the marriage broke up. We simply just grew apart.

Fly:

It was your Ego that got in the way again. You never let your wife see the true person you were, because you didn't know who you were back then. You lived in your own drama as an actor/ bodybuilder/salesman and lived with a lot of people around at all times.

Mansfield

My wife was a person that was conditioned by a big family with lots of cousins and aunts and uncles. She grew up with people all around. The more people, the better. Her Ego would get too bored and insecure with only one person around. She was a person who didn't like to talk about feelings. I didn't want to either, so fourteen years of marriage with no real intimate conversations about how we felt was ok for Ego at the time. She was constantly making friends on vacations, day trips, pool halls, concerts. I could count on one hand the number of times we spent alone on a date together without inviting someone else along. We even had another couple go on our honeymoon with u. Her Ego needed many people around to feel secure. That's how she was conditioned.

Our self likes solitude and just one soul to trust with all the luggage and feelings to feel secure. We were opposites that attracted, burned and then fizzled. It was what it was and I am grateful for all the great experiences. She is a wonderful woman, great mother and will always be my friend.

Florida, Forklifts, a Smile....and a lot 'a Cars

Mansfield:

My consciousness began to awake first around the time I wanted to move to Florida in 2006. My close friend who my wife and I would spend our weekends partying with decided to move to Florida and open a business similar to the one they owned here.

We decided to follow them down a year later in 2006 if we could. I just had to secure a job.

At the time I was acting professionally and selling industrial packaging for eight years. Things were good. I remember walking through a field with my dog late at night and thinking that I had made it. I was really congratulating myself and patting myself on the back.

I had interviewed in St. Louis for a sales manager's position for a packaging company in Orlando and got the job. The only thing that stood in my way now was immigration.

The short of it was that I didn't get the proper paperwork. My immigration lawyer had made a mistake and the Mexican people were marching against the immigration policies of the United States at the time. It didn't happen. But all the stress caused panic attacks when I was alone self medicating with vodka and marijuana.

When it was all over and we were not going to move to Florida, but were going to continue as usual, all the stress stopped, at least on the moving part of it.

But the Ego kept screaming "failure" in my own head. I knew self didn't want to move to Florida, but Ego would justify everything. Major conflict between Ego and self created panic attacks and fainting spells. Once it was settled and I lived a few days back in the now selling packaging products, the stress started to dissipate and the attacks stopped.

Fly:

This emotional experience and breaking of Ego to the point of physical symptoms to the body, is the first of many awakenings. Once you realized what the panic attacks were and got back to what true self wanted, then all returned to normal. It was the realization that you could control your thoughts and therefore control your emotions.

Mansfield:

I left the packaging industry in 2006 because Ego got bored again. I started a new career selling industrial equipment, mainly forklifts. Selling a new product was exciting for the Ego. I started with a company that had a head hunter out looking for salesmen who would be interested in making a career move. So I took the chance. I had no problem selling forklifts. The sales manager had a different type of personality than me. I felt uncomfortable around him. He gave off an energy that really didn't jell with mine. He was a real numbers guy: methodical, technical and dry. I was the opposite. We were on two different frequencies.

I lasted there a year and a half, then jumped to a competitor's brand and sold forklifts for two more years. I did it as an Egoic decision to show my old manager up. No other reason other than Ego flexing its muscles.

Fly:

Two years later in 2010. It was the week you were let go by the fork lift company and you split up with your second wife. She didn't want to go to counseling and had had enough. You were "on the fence". You could have gone either way. You both knew how different people you really were. It would be too much work to try to put a square in a round hole, so you went your separate ways.

You knew that day would come, because you never gave her a chance to get to know the true you. You knew from the beginning that after the parties were over, you had nothing really in common.

Mansfield:

The funny thing was that after the Florida experience and staring failure in the face, at least in my own Ego's eyes, I survived. This experience of being fired and my marriage ending the same month was one of disbelief, amazement, and confusion. I wasn't worried, panicking or anxious. I was emotionally fine. I knew it was a new beginning. I had been slowly making my way to this point for roughly seven years. Now that time had come. I was on my own again. I had married and divorced before, "No big deal".

I moved in with my parents and began to rebuild my life again. I sold my half of the house to my wife but gave it back to her for support for the kids. I left the house with a *Tragically Hip* CD and a vegetable steamer. The steamer was broken.

Living at my parents as a forty-four year old man lasted three months.

I attended my twenty-five year highschool reunion. It was being held at the old hockey arena where I had played so many years before and scored so many goals. It was May and the ice had long been out of the arena. There I saw many familiar faces, many women, but one who caught my eye as soon as I saw her smiling with her friends. She has the smile I could live with for the rest of my life. I didn't know that then, but her beauty blew me away without even speaking a word to her.

By June we had our first date and the rest is history. I found my best friend and the one I want to give all my luggage and insecurities too. The only woman I have ever trusted with the true me. The person I am now and who I just found for myself.

Fly:

The older you get, and the more experiences you have, you start to realize that money should be a means to an end. Do not worship money for it will be your death.

Mansfield:

I needed to find a job to pay my way. I had sold cars before so why not try again. Those hours were good: 9-3pm or 3-9pm. Working on commission was what I had been doing for the last twenty years. I started selling cars again and it was a breeze. It was like riding a bike after twenty years. The program in my mind was still there, it just needed to be dusted off and played.

The slow winters kept for ample amounts of time to read up on the new consciousness. Eckert Tolle, Deepak Chopra. These books helped me realize that I have been awake all this time, but my Ego has been burying self so as there was only one voice after awhile, the voice of Ego and selfishness.

Fly:

Now self was awakening because it had learned from Ego how to do the physical things, the attitude things, and the way you communicate to achieve a goal. It learned the right tones in your voice to use, the body language and all the roles you have played. Now you are ready to take over and do things your way, knowing Ego will always be there for protection. It is a long process to find true self and embrace it.

Mansfield:

I worked at selling cars for another year and a half. As I awoke, I realized I should do what I love. Be in the physical fitness industry. I loved the gym, lived for workouts and could spend the whole day training people. I had done that since 1991.

I took a job at my gym as a personal trainer. It was one of the most fulfilling jobs I ever had. I could get people in shape in a short amount of time, but that became detrimental to the success of the gym because the person I trained didn't renew the personal training contract because I helped them attain their goals. I didn't make enough money. I was still doing steroids. Small doses for maintenance, as the gym crew would say. No one knew. I have had this secret for twenty-two years now.

It was like I had separate lives. One life I portrayed was a family man, husband, good guy, business man, and the other was bodybuilder trying to be an actor.

Fly:

Slowly things began to fall away. All the anxieties. All the stresses. The things we believed to be wasted energy. Who you really were and who you should be. Your life puzzle was becoming somewhat clearer. As you became more conscious of now and who you really were, you realized that acting wasn't really a passion. You were doing it all for the money and fame that could come with it. You always felt like you were just some guy trying to fool everyone into thinking he is an actor. In your mind you thought everyone would think you were somebody, someone special, different, someone better, like all of the celebrities.

Mansfield:

So I quit acting. It started to interfere with being personal trainer. I really enjoyed working with people to meet their fitness goals. I remember getting BOH's (bursts of happiness) while being engaged in a set with a client who would push him or herself more than they usually would, then see the results and be glad they met their goals. To see how happy they were made it the best job I have ever had because it was the most fulfilling.

Fly:

Yes, most fulfilling, but too much time in the day at odd hours. A personal trainer trains when other people are available. It can make for some long days. You could have six clients a day, each for one hour. They would be spread out all day long. This is where a passion can become a burden. When the passion steals away balance, it becomes a burden over time.

Mansfield:

I didn't like those kinds of days because I could never take care of personal business and balancing family and work became too difficult and stressful.

So I changed careers yet again. I started delivering beer for a local craft beer manufacturer.

Fly:

This is where we awoke and became even more mindful. Driving truck, delivering kegs and cases of beer to stores and local businesses has enabled us to realize truth. While comparing notes from Freud, Jesus, and our own experience with physical fitness and bodybuilding we began to connect mind, body and soul.

The Ego was re-conditioned mostly on this job. As awakening was taking place all old Egoic thinking has, and still is, being reconditioned to adapt to the new way of thinking.

This new way of thinking is simply "It is what it is, it was what it was, and it will be what it will be".

You can't change anything about the past and the future hasn't come yet, so don't react emotionally to preserve the even flows of energy passing through the body. Live in truth and excellence by conditioning Ego to be disciplined to always prepare and grow with integrity.

Through this we are always becoming more and more aware. The Eckert Tolle books we read five years ago are all becoming a lot clearer. We have been searching for answers for so long.

Mansfield:

I started to read the bible looking for answers and trying to find similar teachings on the science side of things.

Fly:

Science is a creation of the Ego to define and label what is.

Mansfield:

The cool thing about it was when I started to think about all the experiences I have had over my life, they seem to be melding together for some kind of purpose down the road.

I had asthma as a kid and still do.

Having to come back to the moment and concentrate on every breath made me more in the now all through my life. There were times within the journey that I was very self centred, but I would always have to come back "now" when I had an asthma attack. I believe this is how I am able to remember so much of my past, because I was able to truly come back to the moment when necessary.

From my studies of Freud and Pavlov, I started to see similarities in the parables that Jesus spoke of and the way he taught about controlling Ego.

Fly:

It is fascinating to follow what Jesus taught. In my opinion he was teaching health of the body. He was a therapist for people. He could have been able to manipulate energy through his body to heal people. This might have been possible by being able to activate different parts of his brain through control of thought. We believe that Jesus had no Ego, so he didn't ever have any stress. This is what he was teaching. If you have no stress, your body can function as it should and mind, body and soul live as one.

Jesus taught to be in the moment because it is God's will what happens. Don't react to life, respond to life and the body will prosper with good health.

Scientifically and logically that makes sense, because stress hormone levels would be very low, therefore the body does not have to process excessive amounts of negative cortisol which affect immune system.

Mansfield:

There is another aspect to create the mind, body and soul connection. The body needs to be in good physical shape to make all three aspects whole. You can't ignore one. You can't ignore your vessel.

You need to have a strong set of core muscles and need to be physically active everyday for optimum health.

Doctors these days are trained to treat patients through pharmaceuticals. Pharmaceuticals make money. Pharmaceuticals companies don't want you to be cured. They want to alleviate the symptoms and make them go away while you're on their drug.

Fly:

The body and mind can heal almost all illnesses. The Ego is the obstacle to optimum health. Control the Ego, control your health.

Mindfulness of a Fly on the Wall

This Life, Findings and Observations

Mansfield:

Delivering beer for an hourly wage in 2012, was the first job that wasn't a commission-based job since I was twenty-four years-old. I was now forty-six. I took the job because I liked the physical aspect of lifting 175lbs kegs of beer up and down stairs in the depths of Toronto bars and restaurants. It would supplement my workouts. I wanted a job I could leave and not have to think about and stress over, like the sales jobs I had. I was still taking steroids and justified them with the job.

Fly:

Logic through Ego decided that you had been on them for so long that you would have to stay on low doses for the rest of your life. You had heard of others having heart attacks from coming off steroids and the body not being able to produce enough testosterone to enable the heart to function properly. You had never been to a doctor to check. You were still holding on to that Ego part of your mind. Ego was justifying the steroids to supplement the heavy lifting you did all day long. You were still insecure. Ego's insecurity wouldn't let go.

Mansfield:

I can remember justifying the continuation of the steroids, by starting to compete in bodybuilding again at age 47, in the master's category, age 40-50yrs old. I was still a bodybuilder, still training every day, always making sure I never missed a scheduled day, other than emergencies or sickness. I was lifting beer kegs all day, four days a week, for my job. Ego's logic says continue to take them. At this time in my life, the doses were small at 200-400mg of testosterone every two weeks. It kept my muscles full and it wasn't overkill. It was a maintenance thing. I believed I needed steroids to survive, so I wouldn't have a heart attack.

Being a truck driver teaches you a lot about yourself and your Ego. Driving in downtown Toronto in a twenty-five-foot cube van teaches you something. This is where I began to witness the transformation of my energies and health.

When I started the job, it was a tremendously stressful job, carrying a load of beer, sometimes thirty kegs and one hundred cases, in downtown traffic, and jostling pedestrians.

On my third week on the job, I "doored" a bike rider. That is when you open your car door to an on-coming bike rider by mistake. He was ok health wise, but I got a $120 fine. These things I never worried about in sales, because I was always in industrial areas, with few pedestrians and no bike riders. It can be a stressful job if you are unaware, as I was when I started.

I remember when I started this job how uptight I used to get anticipating a slow, long delivery, not being able to find parking close enough. I would expect the worst all day long. I would swear at other drivers, get stressed out because I had so many deliveries and not enough time. A very stressful mindset.

I soon realized that the more I let go, the easier everything became. The more I worried about the next delivery, the worse it became. So, I stopped worrying, stopped anticipating. I just let it happen. I started to respond, instead of react, to each day. Once I started to do that, I slept better, I trained better, I had way more energy and my mind was clearer. The days would fly by as if time had sped up. Most of the day was spent in alpha consciousness figuring life out. The calmer I stayed, the easier the day was. Even if I had some old conditioning come back to try and trip me up, I consciously would come back to the moment and realize that every night I would end up at home with my family and all would be well.

Fly:

You, we, stopped our old conditioning. Stopped complaining, stressing, trying to control it all. You have to be humble to find the true meaning of it. This is what Jesus was teaching. There will be good days and not so good days, but still in all they will be good. That is what the mind should be living. Then, and only then, will Ego be controlled. Control Ego and control the energy that the body receives around it.

Mansfield:

As time moved on, competitions kept me in control of Ego. I trained hard and became aware that emotions effect cortisol levels. Cortisol is detrimental to building muscle, so every time I found myself in a stressful situation, I began to just respond logically, rather than emotionally.

When I did that consistently, I found I slept better and workouts had a better connection with the muscle. I held on to more muscle preparing for a show by not reacting to everyday life.

Fly:

Cortisol or stress feeds poor health by destroying immune efficiency. It affects sleep, appetite and the ability to think clearly and focus. Remember stress is individually manufactured by the Ego and your conditioning.

Being aware of these things we began to re-condition ourselves. We began to be able to control cortisol through response and not emotional reaction.

Mansfield:

Once we were able to have some control over Ego, our insecurities started to fall away. Once we realized that nothing really matters but right now and that now is all we have and all we ever had, it became easier. Life was starting to become easier.

The more mindful or aware we become, the more we don't need the old Egoic reinforcements that we were so conditioned to search for, that Abraham Maslow spoke of. Life has been simplified and flows like a steady river.

Fly:

We find as Ego and self begin to merge together as one, our old ways of entertaining Ego have drifted away as we find those things and activities to be too boring for Ego.

"Been there done that scenario."

We are more in the moment and do not need to be entertained anymore. We can sit in peace and just be. Meditation is becoming more and more a part of our lives.

We no longer need the steroids because they were all associated with the mask from the old conditioning.

Mansfield:

It has been two years since our last 200mg of testosterone.

The difference from being on steroids and not, is twenty pounds of bodyweight. Strength is down twenty-five percent as we were on them so long. At least twenty-eight years.

Fly:

The steroids are gone and we don't even miss them. We are free.

The workout intensity and frequency has actually stayed the same. Endurance is down twenty percent, which makes sense, with twenty percent less bodyweight given 15lbs was muscle. This means less fuel stored in muscle bellies creates muscle failure sooner. More and more cardio exercise is included these days. It just makes you feel better.

Mansfield:

Steroids were our biggest skeleton in the closet. No one knew, or at least I convinced myself that they didn't know. I never changed my mask, always lifting, always muscular. When I tried to come off for good, people would notice and say "Still working out?" or "Have you lost weight?"

Fly:

Ego hated weakness; Ego wants to be different. Ego wants to be unique. Ego is an insecure child afraid everyone will find out how flawed and weak you are. Ego would always come up with an excuse to do another cycle. Until one day self had enough and decided to evolve to the next level of personal growth.

We quit after the last bodybuilding show and haven't even thought of going back. Now your consciousness is melding with Ego. It is new and wonderful things are happening within. Our personal relationship with nature, the body, and the mind is evolving. The way our conscious is awakening is like a dimmer switch being slowly turned up to bring light in the room.

Yes, Ego always wants more until the realization that Ego will never be satisfied. This is when true self finds a better way.

Mansfield:

Yes, it used to drive us crazy when someone mentioned we looked small or questioned if we were still training. Before long we would hit another cycle. All because that is the mask we decided to don all those years ago. The mask of a bodybuilder. It was created to protect and survive from being bullied. We had been too insecure to find another mask. In the end there will be no masks. Just us, as we are, as we will be, ever evolving ever changing. Now it is one day at a time, live in the moment, enjoy now, be grateful for yesterday and don't worry for it is always "as it should be."

Fly:

After reviewing Freud and Maslow's theories and studying the teachings of Jesus, you relate Ego with the journey to self actualization, as I believe Jesus was, logically. If you connect the three different sources of information on human behaviour with human consciousness, it serves as a guideline for the ability to handle the different energies of the universe through optimum health, to promote mind, body and soul, as one.

Mansfield:

Now, I am starting to see the big picture of my life. My puzzle is coming together nicely. The Fly has opened my mind to new ways of thinking, since the Fly and I have been communicating. It has been seven years now. Life has taken a turn for the better. I feel content, at peace, and physically strong. The clarity of my life puzzle is visible now, but I have always known what it was, just had to get over my conditioning and be my true self.

The Fly doesn't have to argue with me anymore, he just whispers in my ear once in a while to bring me back to the moment. He is actually driving the vessel now with all the knowledge and experience Ego has acquired. He is always there, knowing what the correct thing for me to do is, because of all the life experiences I have had over fifty-one years.

I realize now that the Fly that kept talking to me all my life was really my true self, trying to communicate to my giant Ego, who would not listen to that weaker voice inside.

In actual fact, "The Fly" stayed behind the curtain and knew he would one day take over driving the vessel, watching and learning from Ego, who would eventually become the voice in the background, behind the curtain, always there to help if needed.

I am so thankful for every experience I ever had, I see they are all intertwine, layer upon layer as a lesson or a hint to something that might come. It could be years down the road, but it is all related and if you can see the signs, you can be aware to make the right choices for yourself. You will be able to make choices that will be beneficial to mind, body and soul, as one.

My experiences have made me who I am today and I like what I have become. All we have is now and now is a gift from God. We are now. God is always the energy now. We are all God.

Fly;

You got it man! Take this and realize, Fly out!

I Am, The Fly, Now

Mansfield:

I am the Fly, I am the true self and I am now the driver of this ship. I know what I like and don't like and I am Mansfield Grey.

I realize now that I have always had my Fly on the wall, because I have always felt all my experiences in life were of me watching myself in a movie. I have gone down my Ego's way and realize Ego can never be satisfied.

I realize that I know nothing, but I remember all the experience. I draw from those experiences to respond unemotionally to any conflict that will come my way. I am in control of my emotions to better my health every day.

My goal in life now is that of someone who is not chasing any monetary goal or material item, but that of a soul who seeks knowledge with spiritual peace. I chase balance in life and practise living in the moment as much as possible. I have bursts of happiness (BOH) daily and live for each day as if it were my last. I am truly happy helping others discover their own Fly and their own mindfulness.

I now find that I am more content to just be, instead of having to entertain Ego, all the time. I find meditation has become a normal part of my day. The more aware of old conditioning and Ego, the better my immune system becomes. I become healthier.

My Ego will always be there, but knowing what it is helps to have Ego and self work together for a common goal which is health.

Mindfulness of a Fly on the Wall

Mansfield Truths:

The connection with nature, God and the moment should always be first.

Balance mind, body and soul through discipline of sleep, nutrition, fitness, hydration and consciousness.

Be aware of your own Ego and conditioning, to manage your health.

Always be prepared.

Listen to your intuition, it is the holy spirit that we all have.

Control emotion. Respond, don't react.

With the determination to pursue perfection, evolves excellence.

Live in excellence (D.I.P.) at all times and excellence becomes the norm.

One foot in alpha as much as possible.

Live with integrity and live free!

THE END

For news about future Mansfield Grey stories, join the mailing list at: books@sunaopublishing.com. Please place "Fly" in the subject line.

ABOUT THE AUTHOR

Mansfield Grey *believes the main reason for mental illness in adolescents and young adults has to do with the conditioning and programming of their mind and body. Mansfield wants to help young adults find a better way. The realization of Mansfield's transformation of awareness has led him to self-actualization, through a mind, body spiritual journey that is clearly defined and shows a guide to those individuals that are looking for a better way. Along with re-conditioning of the mind, Mansfield writes of physical re-conditioning to bring all three levels of self awareness together as mind, body and soul, as one, connect with nature.*

*****Stephen Gregory Brown** *(Mansfield's alter Ego) has made the journey to mind, body and soul and has chosen to share that experience with others who may be struggling with their own mindfulness.*

Stephen has been a bodybuilder, professional actor and tradesman. He is the founder of **Nero Gravity Resistance Training** *and teaches its fundamentals to his students.*

Stephen Gregory Brown

Made in the USA
Middletown, DE
27 September 2018